STEPS ALONG THE WAY

A memoir of 13 years
of medical missionary work
in Rhodesia/Zimbabwe

DICK STOUGHTON

LORETTA STOUGHTON

We dedicate this book to all the wonderful Mission and Hospital staff (and many others) who we met and worked with during our missionary work.

PROLOGUE

The longest day—and the longest week—of my life began with a man running into the clinic and saying, "Doctor come quick. There's been an accident." Before that instant, my life had been terrific: a loving wife, four adorable but active boys between four-months and five years, a job I loved, and enough money to pay the bills. I was a Naval Flight Surgeon at Barbers Point Naval Air Station, Oahu, Hawaii. We lived in comfortable Navy housing, the weather was perfect, and the beach called us on many sunny days. Life was good.

As our second year in Hawaii began, I had some extra vacation. An ad by a doctor on the Island of Kauai seeking someone to work in his office for three weeks while he went to California on vacation caught my eye. It was a chance for me to make extra money and still have a working vacation on "The Garden Island." Arrangements were made, we found a small vacation-rental cottage, and the doctor let me use one of his cars. After introducing me to his office staff and explaining the ins and outs of his practice at both the office and the hospital, he gave me the keys to the car and was off, and I was on my own. For a week, everything was as grand as I had expected—the practice was demanding but exciting. While I worked, Loretta and the kids frolicked on a sandy beach of a nearby river; I played golf with the doctors' friends; and one evening we hired a babysitter to look after the kids while we sumptuously dined on mahi-mahi at a beachfront restaurant, soft Hawaiian music accompanied by the soothing sound of crashing surf in the background. Over a glass of wine, I said, "Maybe some day we can do this when I get out of the Navy. Why not live in Hawaii, especially here on the Garden Island of Kauai?"

"Why not? I could do it, if you can find a good practice, but I wouldn't want you to be alone and on call all the time."

" No, I wouldn't do it unless I could be in a group of two or three."

1

The day before that darkest day of my life, Loretta became seriously ill with stomach flu. She was dizzy and vomiting and could barely get out of bed. Since it was my afternoon off, I was able to watch the kids. The next day it was obvious she wasn't going to be able to care for them. I felt I had to be at the office—that's what I was getting paid for. We asked if there was someone who might be able to babysit the three oldest boys, and were referred to a lady who lived only five minutes from our cottage. I don't remember her name—maybe because my subconscious wants it suppressed—but to give her substance, I'll call her Terry. We called Terry and arranged to visit her. They lived on a small hill overlooking the ocean, and in the middle of their huge lawn stood an empty swimming pool. We expressed concern about the pool, wondering aloud if one of our boys might fall into the depth and be injured? The woman reassured us, "I've frequently looked after other children. There's never been a problem."

When we arrived the next morning, the pool was full of water. Terry said, "We felt it would be better to have it full. Then you don't have to worry about one of the kids falling onto the cement."

"I don't know. It worries me. It means you really have to watch *all* of them *all* of the time."

"Trust me. I'll do that."

"Chris is very active so you can't let him out of your sight."

"I won't. Don't worry. Loretta, you go home and take care of the baby and get a good rest."

With reservations, we left the three boys with Terry, I took Loretta home, went to the hospital and then to the office. At 10:30 the man ran into the office with his ominous message. The most horrible thoughts immediately flashed through my mind, all of them involving the pool and one or more of my boys. I ran out of the clinic to my car, but he wouldn't let me drive because he knew I was too upset. As he drove, I stared out the window thinking, "*Why did I leave them with her? I could have taken the day off. The doctor wouldn't have been happy, but that's what I should have done. Something really bad has happened if they're calling me away from work. The pool; one of the boys; why did I leave them with her; where is Loretta?"*

An interminable fifteen minutes later we pulled into the driveway. An ambulance was near the pool, and several people surrounded an EMT who was trying to resuscitate 2-year-old Chris. Loretta ran to me crying, "Oh Dick, he's drowned. They've been working on him for a long time, but no response."

Fiercely holding her, we walked over to where Chris was lying. The EMT looked up at me and shook his head. "I've been doing all I can, Doc, but no response. His pupils are fixed and dilated, no heart beat, no breath. Nothing."

I knelt down to touch and look at Chris. He was cold, blue, and already starting to get stiff. Looking at Loretta, I sobbed and gasped, "He's gone." Standing up to hold onto her, I said to the EMT, "You can stop. I know he's dead."

In 1965 there were no advanced medical procedures for trying to bring drowning victims "back to life." None of my training was of any value. As sad as it was, I knew there was nothing more to do. I couldn't save my own son.

Terry came to us crying, and said, "I was feeding them lunch and suddenly didn't see Chris. I ran right here and saw him in the bottom of the pool. I dove in, got him out, and called emergency." Shaking her head sadly she said, "I can't understand how it happened. I'm so sorry." The rest is just a blur: Explaining to our boys that Chris was dead; flying back to our home near the Naval Station; friends coming to give their condolences; flying to my parents home in Iowa with the body of Chris; a wake, a funeral, and burial in Iowa; some time to recover from the tragedy. But, one never really recovers, do they? Life is changed forever. The very deep gut-wrenching pain slowly wanes but never completely leaves.

For many couples, such an event tears them apart. They start to ask questions like, "Is there really a God? If so, why would He allow this to happen? What have I done to deserve this? How do we handle this? *Why us?*" Some of those penetrated our minds and bounced around like Ping-Pong balls, but not for long. To me, the only question was, "Why did I allow them to stay there when I had reservations? Why didn't I look at that pool and say, 'I'll stay home and take care of them,' but no, I thought it was too important to fulfill my duties at the hospital and office. Why?" No answers, but feeling guilty didn't help. Faith was the answer. *We found that by supporting each other and having faith in each other and faith in God, that somehow, someway, things would work out for us and we would get through this tragedy.*

Our Faith Journey took many turns and stumbles after Chris' death, but gradually, four years later, it led us to the point where we decided to do medical missionary work in Rhodesia from 1970 to 1975, and then after my retirement from a medical practice in Wisconsin, to return to Zimbabwe (formerly Rhodesia) from 2001 to 2009. At the time we made the decision to go to the missions, Loretta had just delivered our sixth child. Mission Doctors Association—the organization we've been associated with for 45 years—told us their "limit" for accepting families for overseas mission work was "five children." *If* Chris had still been alive, would they have accepted us? I don't know. Maybe they would have, but I always felt that Chris was up there helping direct us towards the kind of life God wanted from us—one of service. I know that going to Rhodesia with our family of five children, and returning with seven, was the best thing we ever did. It made us closer as a family and all of us were enriched by the experience. Chris would have loved it, but we believed he was always a big part of us and was enjoying it right along with us.

As I wrote this story, I found that many of the same emotions returned as on the day it happened. In telling others the story, I still have trouble getting through without tears in my eyes. The death of a child is the ultimate tragedy and one never really "gets over it." We're not supposed to bury our children. I truly think that because of the way Loretta and I handled it, we were better people and better as a married couple. I also think it made me a more compassionate doctor with more empathy for people, especially those who lost a child. In Rhodesia in the 1970s, many children died of preventable diseases like measles and whooping cough. Because of the frequency of the deaths, I became a bit hardened to them—it was just too difficult to go through the emotional rollercoaster of children dying day after day. However, because of my empathy, I resolved to initiate a campaign to vaccinate all the children in our District, and instead of treating hundreds of sick children—many of whom would die—we would get out of the hospital and into the community to immunize them. We accomplished it and saved hundreds of lives as a result. Chris lives on in our memories—we don't talk about him much, but he's still there. Our Catholic Faith teaches us that children dying at that age go directly to heaven. I believe that, so when I'm wanting some special favor from God it's not unusual for me to pray to our own Saint Christopher: "Dear Chris, please intercede for me, and ask God to grant me the grace to get through this difficult time."

It works.

A *Step Along the Way* is our story of that missionary journey.

PROLOGUE #2

I have been told that to write a successful memoir, one must either be famous or infamous, or at least have a story with sex or addiction (or preferably both) or violence or severe conflict or humor or suffering or an internal struggle or conversion or I don't know what else. This story doesn't have any of the above. Sure, there are conflicts and struggles, but it's mostly a story about a missionary couple's experiences while working with the very poor in Rhodesia/Zimbabwe, between 1970 and 2009. We loved the people and the work and hope that you will see that love as you read our story.

CONFLICT

"Mai Wei! Mai Wei! Mai Wei!" ("Woe is me! Woe is me! Woe is me!) wailed the mother, as she threw herself onto the cement floor and crying and howling and pounding her fists, then howling some more. I stood by helplessly. What could I do? How should I react to such a gut-wrenching display of anguish? Sister Anne Marie, having seen it many times, knelt beside the heartbroken woman, quietly talking and cooing as though consoling a small child. After many minutes of pounding the cement and shouting "Mai Wei" over and over, the crying slowly ceased and she weakly stood and said, "Torai ini ku murumbwana wangu (Take me to my son)."

To me it felt like the beginning of the end of my brief career as a medical missionary in Rhodesia. Having arrived just six weeks before, I thought I was slowly learning about working in this totally foreign environment—foreign language, foreign conditions, foreign feeling of being mostly alone in making medical decisions. Now I had made a decision, and it was the wrong one. Her child was dead, and he died because I attempted to do something I shouldn't have done.

It started on a quiet Saturday morning at our home on Driefontein Mission in rural Rhodesia, in August 1970. Did I say quiet? Mike and Tom were fighting over who got to work on a model airplane, Doug and Mary were screaming at each other because Mary had a toy Doug wanted, Paul was crying because he wanted attention from someone, the dog was barking because of all the noise, and I was reading and listening to Rachmaninoff, fairly oblivious to the commotion. Loretta came in and said, "Can't you do something about this noise?"

"Huh? Sorry, I didn't even hear them," I replied. When I'm reading, I can tune out the world—it's the only way I got through medical school.

Exasperatedly she said, "Take these wild kids outside and play with them. I need them out of my hair so I can get some work done today."

Just then the phone rang. A nurse from the hospital said, "Good morning doctor. How are you today?" — an African[1] *always* greets you before saying anything else, no matter what the emergency.

"I'm fine. How are you?"

"I'm fine. Doctor, we have a five-year-old boy who swallowed a rivet, and is having trouble breathing. Please come right away."

"I'll be right there."

"Sorry, dear. I've got to go. Emergency at the hospital."

She rolled her eyes and sighed, "I know."

I rode my bike down the dirt road, past the eucalyptus forest and the 300-bed Tuberculosis Sanatorium and another mile to the general hospital, thinking, "*I wonder if he inhaled that rivet. I hope not.*" Little did I know it was the beginning of a story I'd rather forget.

As soon as I walked into the outpatient department, I knew the boy was in serious trouble because I could hear him wheezing from the corridor. As I entered the exam room, he was struggling to take a breath. With wide eyes he looked from his father to me as if to say, *Do something quick*. An x-ray showed a metallic foreign body in the right lower lung. Not something he swallowed, but something he inhaled and it "went down the wrong way," right to the bottom of the right bronchiole tube. Through an interpreter, the

---

1   A note on the language used here. When we were in Rhodesia during the 1970s, the government and society recognized 3 categories of people that had specific laws regulating them. "Whites or Europeans" were the Caucasian population of mostly European ancestry who had the most privilege; "Blacks or Africans " were those of indigenous African ancestry, and had the fewest rights and most persecution; "Colored" were people of Arab, West asian, or mixed ancestry, and had more rights than the Blacks and less than the Whites. I use this vernacular in this memoir, as that was the vernacular used by the entire population during the events being described.

father said, "Tatenda was sucking on a small metal rivet this morning, and suddenly started coughing. We live nearby and came right away."

The x-ray looked like a metal rivet—very small, like a tiny pawn on a chess set. It wouldn't be easy to remove. I told the father, "You'll have to take him to Salisbury (120 miles away). I know it's far, but the boy needs a specialist to remove the tiny rivet."

"No, I can't go there. It's too far."

"You must. We can't do it here. It's too difficult and dangerous."

"I'm afraid to take him so far from home. If they operate and he dies, his spirit won't find its way home." During my time in Rhodesia I learned this belief in the persons' spirit after death is very important in the decision making process for most Africans. It might even be more important than saving one's life. They believe it's imperative for the spirit to be able to find its way back to their original home. Otherwise it will wander around for years and years and cause problems for family members that remain behind—in other words, they might become "bewitched." If there's a possibility the person might die, they will opt for dying close to home, even if there would be a better chance to live if they went to the large hospital in Salisbury.

"You must take him to Salisbury."

"I can't. If you don't treat him, I'll take him to the n'anga (witch-doctor or traditional healer)." It was obvious to me the boy would probably die if the rivet wasn't removed. He already was in respiratory distress. I again tried to convince him to go to Salisbury.

He refused, saying, "Do what you can." Over the next several years I heard the same statement over and over, and each time it left me with a sense of "Why me? Why do I have to take the risk?" But of course, it wasn't me but the patient who was taking the risk. In this case, the father was assuming the risk for his son.

"What do you think, Sister Anne Marie?" She was the anesthetist on-call that day, a diminutive German Dominican Nun who was the Matron (Head Nurse) of the hospital. Although weighing barely 100 pounds, she had an iron will. No one on the staff tried to cross her. I had watched her over the previous six weeks while she managed staff and student nurses. I'd seen her stand toe-to-toe with a very large staff nurse and let her know in no uncertain terms that she *would* do it the right way or she could look for a new job. On the other hand, I'd also observed her when she was kind and loving with a staff member who had personal problems. Competent, compassionate, firm, and usually quiet.

Speaking in Shona, she spoke animatedly with the father, but he kept shaking his head indicating that "No, he would not take him to Salisbury. No way."

Turning to me she said, "I think if we don't treat Tatenda, he'll take him to the witchdoctor and then he'll have no chance. We see this a lot, and because of it, we feel forced to do things we'd rather not do. I think we should try to get the rivet out and I believe you can do it."

We both recognized the difficulty on such a small boy. "What other options do we have?" I asked.

"I don't see any. It's risky, but doing nothing means he'll probably die."

I was struggling with the idea of *me* trying to remove the rivet. On the one hand, I appreciated her trust in my abilities, and I was confident enough to think that with proper attention to anesthesia, I could remove it. On the other hand, if something went wrong and there were complications, I could justifiably be criticized for attempting something beyond my ability. Because *something* needed to be done, I decided to go ahead. How I wish I hadn't.

Sister put the boy to sleep, making sure he was well ventilated with oxygen. I took the rigid metal bronchoscope tube and inserted it through his mouth, through the voice box, and down the right main-stem bronchus. The rivet was at the bottom of the bronchus, glistening black inside the pink bronchus, so small and smooth. I carefully inserted thin forceps down to the rivet, but couldn't grasp it. I could see it, but it was too slippery and the forceps kept sliding off the rivet. It was taking too much time.

"I need to give him oxygen," said Sister Anne-Marie. I removed the 'scope just seconds before I could grasp the rivet and she gave him oxygen for a few minutes. "O.K. You can try again."

We went through this scenario several times and each time when she became concerned, she would let me know and I would remove the 'scope so she would give more oxygen. As I tell this story today, we have to remember there were no such things as oxygen saturation monitors or even heart monitors back then, so the only way she could judge was by listening to the heart beat, and noting his color—not so easy in a small dark-skinned boy.

I realize now that during the final time, when at last I got the rivet, it had taken too much time. He had a cardiac arrest, maybe due to the final stimulus of pushing the forceps hard against the rivet to grasp it. No heart beat as I removed the rivet. I used all the resuscitation skills I learned during my residency to revive him. We worked feverishly for more than an hour, but to no avail. With deep sadness I had to tell the parents that Tatenda was dead.

The parents wanted to see their son, so we took them into the operating room. Still lying on the operating table, he looked so small and innocent, but also so lifeless—to me. The mother gasped, touched his cold body, and only then fully realized he was indeed dead. With a loud cry, she again threw herself onto the cement floor in such a way that I was sure she must hurt herself. The keening and wailing and pounding of her fists on the floor seemed to go on forever. Then, as if a record had reached its end, she abruptly stopped crying, stood, put her son on her back, securing his body in place by wrapping a large towel around both of them, and with her husband alongside, they started for home. As she approached other people near the hospital, the wailing started all over again. I could hear the sad moaning until it gradually decreased as she walked farther and farther from the hospital and finally faded to nothing but the afternoon wind.

How many times in the years to come would I hear that same outpouring of grief? Each time a chill would go down my spine, partly because it brought me back to the moment when this woman showed me how the death of her son had torn her heart apart. I would stand by helplessly, not knowing what to do other than to be quiet and supportive. Each time I would be there to answer questions *if* there were any, and to help with whatever papers had to be completed. Each time I would feel defeated.

Although our first six weeks of learning to do this "medical missionary thing" had been overwhelming and at times disorienting, nothing compared to this. Why did I agree to do the procedure? What do I do now? Not wanting to go home in such an emotional state, I rode my bike aimlessly around the mission. Watching the parents with their dead child reminded me of the time, six years earlier, when Chris died. I remembered that kick-in-the-gut hurt that we thought might never go away, and I knew these parents now suffered those same terrible feelings.

I slammed the bike down and collapsed to the ground under a jacaranda tree. *Why did this happen? Why are we here? Is this really what God has called us to do? Why did I ever agree to do that procedure? Was I too proud and overconfident? Was it poor judgment? It's like asking the really big questions: "Why do bad things happen? Why do good people die, and especially such a young child?" How do I get my arms around this tragedy? What effect will it have on my ability to do my work? Will people think I'm incompetent and not want to see me? Am I incompetent? Why do I feel sorry for myself when it's the parents who are suffering?* I listlessly stared at the horizon. No answers. *WHY are we here, God? WHY did you call us to do this work?*

Our journey to Rhodesia was a convoluted one, as are many "faith journeys." After serving my time in the U. S. Navy, I completed a Family Practice residency in California, and we moved to a small town in the foothills of Colorado, thinking it was where we were going to spend the rest of our lives. The medical partnership situation didn't work out, and the result was that we soon started talking about "where do we go from here?" One evening, after putting the boys to bed, we were sitting in the back yard, enjoying a non-alcoholic beer — Loretta was eight months pregnant — and pondering our future. I turned to Loretta and said, "It looks like we're definitely going to move. You may think I'm crazy, but I've always thought we might do medical missionary work when I retired. Now I'm wondering if God might be telling us the time is now. What do you think?"

Surprise of surprise, with a huge smile on her face, she answered, "Dick, I've always wanted to do missionary work, but didn't say anything because I thought you were too practical to consider it."

I should have realized that would be her response, even with the delivery of our sixth child so imminent. She had followed me through three moves in Omaha; then to Oakland, California for my Internship; to Pensacola, Florida for Flight Surgery training; to my Navy assignment in Hawaii for three years; to Santa Rosa, California for my two-year residency; and finally to Colorado where we were going to "settle forever and ever and not have to move again." It seemed another child was born at each location—two in Omaha, one in Oakland, one in Hawaii, one in Santa Rosa, and soon one in Colorado. Never complaining, always ready to see what the next adventure might be. With her statement about "always wanting to do missionary work" as the stimulus, we soon contacted Mission Doctors Association in Los Angeles. The day after Paul was born, I flew to L.A. to be interviewed by MDA Board Members, and we were accepted into that years' mission preparation class.

We informed our families about this sudden change in our life plans. It was one thing for us to live across the ocean in Hawaii—they were happy to visit us there—but quite another to live in "darkest Africa" where there would be all kinds of unknown hazards and no chance to visit. Right from the beginning we knew we would be going to Rhodesia, because that was where the need was most critical. "Do you really *need* to do this?" "Why do this now when you finally have your license and can open an office and make a good living?" "It just seems so far away and we won't see any of you for another three years," were just some of the comments. Of course, there was worry in their voices as we discussed our plans, but they gradually accepted that this was important to us, and then encouraged us to do what we thought was best.

Six weeks later, we handed the house keys to the realtor, walked out the front door, and headed for Los Angeles. The day before, I loaded the Ford Station Wagon with boxes of clothes and books, with just enough room for four kids and me. I told Loretta, "We look like Ma and Pa Kettle heading west." There still was a mountain of boxes of dishes, kids toys, games, and all that junk we think we absolutely must have to survive, and I carefully packed those into our Open Road Camper, hoping they wouldn't fall and create a mess if Loretta had to suddenly stop. On the two-day trip, we would sleep in a motel and eat at restaurants, which was fine with Loretta. She drove the camper, taking infant Paul with her, so she could stop and breast-feed him whenever necessary. People said we were impulsive and adventurous, but we felt we had a calling to do something more with the talents God gave us. Maybe the situation not working out in Colorado was just a way for God to get our attention. Missionary work seemed to be the calling we were hearing, so we eagerly looked forward to the next chapter in our life—the first of our many steps along the way.

As I sat under that Jacaranda tree reminiscing about how we got to Africa, I realized the idea of working in a Third World Country was in the back of my mind ever since I heard Dr. Tom Dooley speak in 1959 about his work in Laos and Cambodia. He talked enthusiastically and emotionally about the work and the people and the great need for medical care for the poor. As the 400 students, nurses, and doctors walked out of the auditorium on that wintry day in Omaha, there was excited chatter about "I wonder if I could ever do that?" "How can I sign up to help him?" "Does he have a volunteer organization?" Before graduating in 1962, I read his book *The Night They Burned the Mountain*. In it he reminisces about meeting the renowned Dr. Albert Schweitzer on the Ogowe River in West Africa.

Dooley went there to find inspiration and insight on how to move ahead with his work in Asia. Dr. Schweitzer told him: "The significance of a man is not in what he attains, but rather in what he *longs* to attain." Dooley's motivating talk remained in my subconscious mind and eventually served as the basis for me to think maybe, just maybe, I could do something to make a difference in an area where people had little access to medical care—as long as that was the goal I really wanted to attain.

With emotions drained, I headed home. I knew I could talk this over with Loretta, my 5-foot-3-inch black-haired Irish-German lass from South Dakota. Ever since we married in 1959, she has been the compass of my life. Her compass seems to always point to "True North," and whenever mine starts to drift South, she's there to gently (and sometimes not so gently) nudge me back to North.

As I trudged into the house with a hangdog expression on my face, she knew something bad had happened. After eleven years of marriage, she was attuned to my many moods. With a furrowed brow, she asked, "What happened?"

I told her about the boy, about the operation, about him dying, and about how bad I felt. She tried to console me, but really knew I just needed someone to talk to and someone who would listen and not judge. We talked for an hour and I felt better just having her listen to me. It was getting late in the afternoon and she had to get supper ready, so she said, "Go out and play with the kids. They'll help take your mind off this."

"Hey, Dad. Where've you been? We've been waiting to play catch with you all day," said Mike, the oldest. A thin 10-year-old, with a mop of thick black hair and glasses that made him look a bit like Harry Potter, and like Harry, always ready for adventure.

"I had an emergency at the hospital. Now I have time, so get the gloves and ball."

"I want to play too," said Tom, age eight, and never wanting to be left behind.

"Me too, me too," echoed around the field. Tom, Doug, and even three-year-old Mary, thought they should be included in the game. We threw the ball around a bit and then someone got the bat, and it was time for hitting lessons.

"Stand this way," I demonstrated. "Then swing the bat level to hit the ball. Keep your eye on the ball and not the bat." Everyone had a turn, with varying results, and after an hour we were tired and it was time for supper.

"Thanks, Dad," I heard as we walked into the house. I must admit it distracted me from the days' events, but during the night I tossed and turned, saying to myself over and over, *Why did I decide to do it? How can I feel sorry for myself when it's the parents who are suffering so much? What should I have done differently?* The next morning I approached work with many doubts lurking in my unsettled mind.

I hoped to share the experience with Dr. George, my colleague and fellow medical missionary. Although we didn't have what one might call a warm relationship, I still hoped we could at least discuss difficult cases, and maybe he would give me some advice and even a little support. Then again, maybe not.

When I saw Dr. George at the hospital, he already knew about the boy's death. I said to him, "Can I talk with you about this case?"

Without looking directly at me he said, "Well, obviously you shouldn't have attempted it," and walked away. His sharp response cut right through me, and with open-mouthed surprise I watched him go down the corridor. I hoped we could discuss the case. Perhaps he could give the advice and support I was so desperately seeking. He was much older than I, but didn't have the same Family Practice Residency training I did. He learned by experience, and I knew experience is a great teacher. For many years, he was the only doctor in a small town in North Dakota before deciding to do missionary work. I hoped he would have a lot to offer a young doctor like me.

I later wondered if he was somehow jealous or upset with me because of my training? Since he didn't have post-graduate training, did he feel inferior? If he did, why? Had I offended him in some way by not asking for his help? I don't know, but realized from our first week at the Mission, his actions and words showed he didn't like me. It bothered me a lot. What had I done to deserve it? Am I that difficult to get along with? I usually made friends easily and don't have enemies. What happened? Even though he didn't like me, I still hoped we could discuss difficult cases, but now realized it wouldn't happen. Maybe he preferred to be alone and that's why he was in a solo practice in North Dakota? I tried to find the reason for his behavior, but there was no way to effectively communicate. I asked Brother Lucian, the hospital administrator, to help us. That didn't work either. We were like two solo practitioners in a small town who won't work or speak with each other. I wondered what others thought about it? No one said anything to me, but they knew there was tension between us. And we were doing missionary work! *Is this why I'm here, God? To be tormented like this? What kind of example are we giving to others?*

During our mission classes in Los Angeles, we were told there would be days when things would be bleak, and now it sure felt like that. We were also told we would run into personality conflicts which seemed unsolvable. How true. In fact, Monsignor Brouers, the founder of "Mission Doctors

Association," went so far as to say those situations were examples of *how we could grow spiritually*. I didn't feel like growing spiritually. I felt angry and upset and depressed. I felt that instead of spirituality, I needed TLC. *Where do I turn when a colleague spurns me and doesn't give me any space for resolving our conflict?*

I needed to dig deep into my psyche and re-think how I approached work. I wasn't going to be the next Dr. Albert Schweitzer in Africa or the next Dr. Tom Dooley in Asia but I would do the best I could on my own. Loretta and the kids would be my reality and my sanctuary.

A week later, I made another attempt to crack the nut of incompatibility with George. The previous week I had seen him playing tennis with his son on the nearby clay tennis court. It looked like great fun as they hit balls, ran after wide shots, and shouted when they hit a winner. I thought maybe we could capture some of that spirit if we played a few sets.

I'm not very good at tennis, but I like to play and enjoy the exercise. With some trepidation, I went over on a Saturday afternoon and knocked on their back door. George opened it and looked at me suspiciously, saying "Yes?"

"Hi, George. I saw you and your son playing tennis last week, and wonder if you would like to play with me today?"

He stood in the doorway, chewing on a toothpick as he mulled over my request. He looked like he was thinking about how to respond: *Yes, because I can beat him badly; No because I don't want to have anything to do with him.* Finally he nodded yes, and said, "I'll be right there."

Well! He was a very good player and I'm not—he whipped me in three sets, running me from side to side with easy strokes, while I flailed away and barely got the ball over the net, or didn't even get to the ball. If that wasn't bad enough, he obviously enjoyed beating me so easily. Each winning shot was associated with a sly smirk on his face. As I produced one weak serve after another—all of which he sent whizzing past me, and sometimes right at me—I tried not to show my displeasure, but it was difficult. Mercifully, he decided it was enough after beating me six-love in three sets. I walked to the net to shake hands, but he stayed at the baseline glowering. I waved a hand and said, "Nice game George. You're way out of my league, but I enjoyed the exercise. . . I wonder if we could sit and have a beer and discuss what's going on between us?"

"Nope," he said and walked away. Nothing more. No explanation at all. He just walked away to his house. I picked up my racket and the balls and slowly shuffled home, feeling not only whipped in tennis but also in life. So much for an attempt at reconciliation.

As I walked in the door, Loretta asked, "Well, how did the tennis match go?"

"Horrible. He whipped me, and what's worse, he enjoyed it. Then he refused to sit with me, enjoy a beer, and discuss our situation."

Doug looked up, interested in what I was going to say. "Go play outside. I want to talk with your mother." Loretta gave me a hug and said, "I'm sorry. I was so hoping and praying this might be an icebreaker. I know you feel terrible about it. You need to realize you can't control his actions. You can only control the way you react to him. You'll get through it and still do the good work I know you can do."

She knows me well. I'm an eternal optimist by nature and she realized with her support and the rest of the family, I would get through this. If George and I were to continue together for three years, it was going to be a long three years, but I would dig deeper into my well of faith, and as usual, lean on Loretta for all the support she could give. When things are tough like this, she would say, "Let's pray about it. It will all work out." And it would, one way or another. I guess this was one of those steps in my spiritual growth, but it sure felt like two steps backwards.

As I thought back on Dr. Dooley's talk in 1959, and what he wrote in his book, I realized that now that I was "out in the bush" in Rhodesia, I needed to apply some of Dooley's perseverance: learn how to cope with a colleague who didn't like me; how to cope with the myriad of problems of working at a remote hospital with little in the way of supplies and a bare minimum of x-ray and laboratory tests; learn how to treat all of the new (to me) tropical diseases; and how to treat people who didn't speak English and I didn't seem to have the knack for learning Shona.

I thought this missionary work was going to be exciting and fulfilling, but instead it's hard and demanding and the conflict with George is dragging me down and I don't know how to fix it and I don't know if I'll be able to adjust to how I see patients so that I can see my share of the 300 patients at the T.B. Sanatorium and the 100 patients at the general hospital and how do I learn about all of these new tropical diseases and will we ever be able to learn Shona and will Loretta adjust to these living conditions, and. . .

"Hail Mary, full of grace. . ."

Letter from Loretta: *September 9, 1970*

Dear Mom and Dad,

It must be a family failing—putting letters down and finishing them a month later. You are lucky though, our shipment arrived and with it my typewriter, so you won't have to decypher my handwriting. As you can see, it doesn't spell very well. Our shipment came through okay, no damage to anything, but one barrel came open and we lost two basketballs, the sleeves and front and back of a sweater I started years ago (yay), and some Tupperware. I'm amazed at what we brought. We thought we'd be far from civilization for three years, and brought everything we would need. It isn't that way at all. It's just that we are an hour's drive from shopping—everything you could want except for children's toys are available.

Our house is good sized and comfortable. It gets down to freezing in the winter and the only heat we have is the fireplace. We can buy electric heaters if it gets too bad. We arrived on the 4th of July, the middle of winter here, and it was pretty cold the first week, but hasn't been bad since. It's now spring, October and November are supposed to be the worst months as it is hot and muggy. The rains start in Nov. or Dec. and take care of the humidity.

Back to our house: We have 5 bedrooms, (small), one that we use for ironing & sewing, living room, dining room, kitchen, pantry, and bathroom. The 20 year-old stove and fridge work well, but are noisy. We have a nice yard. On the side of the house is a play area—I should say construction area. It's very dangerous to walk through because the children are digging dams and canals and forts. The sand is perfect for them to play in. We have a tennis court nearby. Anthills here are cement hard, and that's what was used.

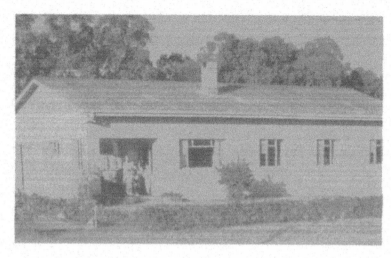

Our Archbishop from Los Angeles was here for a few days. Can you imagine having an Archbishop for breakfast?—lunch and dinner too. I don't have a tablecloth so I used a sheet. He was very nice and we all felt comfortable with him.

In the same area as our house is the African Motherhouse and Novitiate. Around us is a lovely Eucalyptus forest. We are walking distance from the Mission complex to the north, the T.B. sanitarium to the west, and the Regional House for the Bethlehem Fathers and Brothers to the east. The general hospital is a mile down the road beyond the sanatorium.

The Mission includes workshops for carpentry, metalwork, electrical, plumbing, carving, and tailoring, each with schools to teach the Africans those trades. There also is a butchery, dairy, flourmill, and bakery that supplies food for the thousand people living and working at the Mission and the 400 patients in the two hospitals. The hospitals have their own kitchens and laundries, and each has a convent for the Dominican Sisters and for the African Sisters. Imagine, it's the law that Europeans and Africans (even religious) can't live under the same roof! The Bethlehem Brothers also run a farm with a thousand head of cattle, some sheep, pigs, and a large dairy herd. There are orchards with citrus fruit and grapes, some apple and peach trees and a large vegetable garden. Whatever the

Mission doesn't furnish in the way of food, we can charge at a store in Gwelo. Besides all this, we receive $120 a month, so we're very well off!

Mike and Tom are in Gwelo for a few days. Dr. Davies, the government Doctor who is head of TB in this part of the country, has 6 children, with 2 boys exactly Mike and Tom's ages, so we invited them for a week. After 5 days, the 8 year old looked so sad that I had to take them home. Our boys were invited back, so I sent them in with a lorry on Monday. Mike is walking around with pneumonia. We had x-rays taken for a TB check, and discovered that Paul, Doug, and Mike have Bronchial Pnumonia. (I told you this machine couldn't spell). Mike was already gone when Dick checked the results, typical Doctor's family story. I thought something was wrong with Paul, but thought Doug and Mike just had their usual icky nose problem. Anyway they're on the road to recovery now.

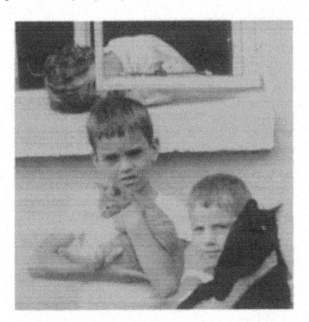

Mary in the window & Tom and Doug holding the cats, at our house Driefontein

Saturday we're invited to visit Silveira Mission. The O'Leary's are there with six children. They have one boy and he is Mike's age. One girl is Mary's age, and when they were here about a month ago, Mary

just moved into the house where they were staying. When they got in their car to leave, she got in too, and when we made her get out, she sneaked back in. They have a large Volkswagen van, in case you were wondering how you could sneak into a car with eight people and four puppies and the mother dog and not be noticed.

Love to all, Loretta

Rhodesia, a land-locked country the size of Montana, located just above the Northern border of South Africa, was named after Cecil Rhodes, the British Empire builder. His company, the British South African Company, obtained mineral rights to the entire area from the most powerful local traditional leaders in 1888, and a charter for BSAC to have exclusive mineral rights was signed by Queen Victoria in 1889. In 1890, a pioneer column of white settlers, led by hunter Frederick Selous, travelled from South Africa through the lightly inhabited countryside and established Fort Victoria at what is now Harare, the capital of Zimbabwe. Of interest is that five Dominican Missionary Nuns (two Irish and three German) were part of the 1890 pioneer column, suffering all the difficulties and hardships of travelling 750 miles in ox-carts, through the wild and mostly unknown territory, crossing rivers, dealing with tropical diseases – especially malaria – and finally reaching Fort Victoria in July 1891. They immediately went to work as nurses at the local hospital, and in 1892 established the first school. They have been operating schools and hospitals in the country ever since.

Two short wars were fought against Matabele warriors, the second ending in 1897, resulting in de facto white rule for the new country of Rhodesia. Because of excellent farmland, many more settlers arrived from England, Germany, South Africa, and Mozambique. The country remained primarily an agrarian economy for many decades. Colonial self-government was allowed by Britain in 1924. Black males were allowed to run for the legislature, but the restrictions on voter eligibility were so strict that few Africans met the qualifications to vote. Inequalities between whites and blacks were established from the beginning, and persisted until Black Independence in 1979. In 1959 the white population became worried about the wave of violence spreading through Africa. The struggle for black rule was spreading and the colonial powers in Europe were looking for ways to bring about change without violence, but without much success. The white colonial settlers throughout the continent were not going to allow such seismic change without a serious struggle. In Rhodesia the white legislature started passing

repressive laws against all African organizations, especially political organizations. In 1960 violence and riots broke out in the large black townships,
resulting in ever more repressive laws. Between 1960 and 1965, more than
1000 blacks were sentenced to prison sentences, many for minor charges
that the white population considered to be treasonous. As a member of the
British Commonwealth, Britain still had significant sway on relations with
the country, and started insisting on more accommodations for the black
political parties. Whites in Rhodesia disagreed, and in 1965 unilaterally
declared complete independence from Britain. Most of the world applied
sanctions to the country, but white-ruled South Africa did not, so normal
world commerce continued via South Africa, and the country prospered —
after a fashion.

Such was the situation when we arrived at Driefontein Mission in
July 1970.

EFFECTING CHANGE?

O ctober 1970, a brisk crystal-clear October morning in Rhodesia—one of those days you're happy to be alive. A Blue-bird day for a pilot. Departing in the Mission owned Cessna 182, I climbed to an altitude of 6500 feet—1500 feet above ground level. Jacaranda trees in full blossom dotted the landscape like purple umbrellas scattered through dull winter fields. The rainy season would start in a few weeks, and none too soon from my standpoint. Since Rhodesia is in the Southern Hemisphere, the seasons are reversed for us Northern Hemisphere dwellers. I was still having difficulty thinking of October as Spring. People assured me the summer rains would soon start, turning the brown farmland verdant green. The mornings were still cool. As I left that morning it was 45 degrees, but soon warmed to the mid-70's.

I was on my way to Kana Mission, a small outlying clinic, for our "Flying Doctors" support. Each month, we flew to eight different clinics, giving those small clinics the medical support they so urgently needed. The few hours per month we spent at each clinic weren't much, but it gave the nursing staff a feeling that someone cared about their work. We hoped our help would make a difference. My predecessor at Driefontein, Dr. Leo Brown and his wife Blue, convinced Mission Doctors Association Auxiliary in Los Angeles to raise money for the Cessna 182 single engine airplane. In 1967, they flew commercially to Cape Town, South Africa to collect the airplane. In five days they studied the South African private pilot rules and regulations, passed both the written and flight tests, cleared the plane through customs, flew it up to Salisbury for Rhodesian clearance, and then to Driefontein where they were instrumental in establishing the Flying Doctors program.

Through it we provided consultation services to a population of more than 100,000 poor black Rhodesians. I love to fly, so this combined two loves: flying and medicine.

Shortly after leaving Driefontein, I flew over several white-owned farms—large estates with rectangles of cultivated land, straight-line fences, and herds of cattle in the winter pastures. There were patches of blue water behind small dams on nearly every farm—water used for irrigation. Each farmhouse was a sprawling affair with large verandahs and green lawns, even in this dry season. Some distance from each main house was a village of African style huts—round, brown mud huts with grass-thatched roofs—at least fifty on each farm, housing the African farm workers. As I flew over, women and children waved and I waggled my wings in response.

Seventy miles later was a different story. The elevation was 2500 feet instead of 5000, meaning it was hotter during the summer. No dams and no water; mostly sandy soil with scraggly bushes and a few huts scattered here and there; a few cattle but many goats. Horrible animals—in my view—because they pull even the slightest tuft of grass from the ground, ruining what could be good pastureland if allowed to rest during the dry season. It was obvious the area was much dryer than the white farms. I could see it was poor agricultural land, with only a few cultivated fields. Once, not so long ago, it was probably good land for wild animals. With the arrival of the white settlers, there slowly but inexorably was a "resettlement" of blacks from good farmland to this arid, bleak landscape. It still looked like it would be better as a game refuge than for farming. But then, that's why these people were called "subsistence farmers"—on this scrubby land, they could barely "subsist." It was not their choice they were trying to farm barren land. The White minority government had placed the "Tribal Africans" on areas that we in America used to call reservations—land not unlike the very poor land in South Dakota where we settled large numbers of Sioux Indians, and with similar results. The White farmers took the choice land where there was sufficient rain and good soil.

Finding Kana Mission Clinic was never easy due to few visual navigational aids along the way. It was mostly by "dead reckoning"—using time and compass direction to figure out where I was and when I should arrive at my destination. I watched for landmarks, but they weren't easy to find, being mostly dried-up rivers. I had been there a couple of times, but always with someone who helped navigate. I was alone and having trouble finding the mission. First I flew up one dry riverbed—no mission; then turned north and found another and flew down that—no mission; turned south and found another one to fly up. I was getting worried I would soon have to admit I was lost and unable to find the mission, when out of the corner of my eye I spotted some low-lying buildings with tin roofs. Kana Mission! Praise the Lord. I made a low pass over the mission to let them know I had arrived, and then flew really low over the grass airstrip to make sure there were no cattle, goats, or new anthills. Anthills could crop up overnight, growing as tall as one to two feet and hard as cement. It would ruin my day if I hit one of them with an airplane wheel at 60 miles an hour. No animals or anthills in sight. Checking the windsock, I realized a moderate crosswind was going to make for a tricky landing. After a standard approach, I floated to a landing, first hitting the left wheel and then the right and bouncing once. Well, that wouldn't get my instructors' approval, but I was safely down. Taxiing to the end of the bumpy runway, I shut down the power. Several small children appeared from nowhere to look at the plane, laughing and giggling, pointing and jabbering in Shona—which I didn't understand, even though we had been taking Shona lessons three evenings a week. So far I was not having much success in understanding what might as well have been Chinese.

Father Joe, one of the Spanish priests from the mission, arrived in a beat-up pickup, along with a young African man. "Hello Doctor. Glad to see you."

"Hello Father Joe. Good to see you. How is everyone here at Kana?"

"As well as can be expected at this time of year. We're anxiously waiting for rain and pray it will be better than last season. Our people are starving."

"Yes, it looks like desert from the air. Nothing in the rivers and no dams in this area."

"Get in and I'll take you to the clinic. This is Patrick. He'll keep an eye on your plane so those scamps don't get too close."

"Thanks," and he drove me the mile to the clinic. Driving onto the Mission grounds was a complete contrast to Driefontein. The buildings were unpainted and in poor repair; there were a few broken windowpanes; goats and chickens everywhere. The main problem was money—they received little support from Spain whereas Driefontein had loads of help from wealthy Switzerland. Even in Mission organizations there are the rich and the poor, and Kana was very poor. Still, they were cheerful people doing God's work in this remote area.

I quickly learned that I first needed to greet everyone. All over Africa, it is very impolite to just "get to work." To all the staff, I would say: "Mangwanani (Good Morning)."

They all answered, "Mangwanani."

I said, "Mamuka Sei? (How did you get up?)" Several of the younger clinic staff snickered and giggled at my pronunciation of Shona words, but I was determined to at least master the words of greeting.

They answered, "Ndamuka kana mamakawo (I got up well if you got up well.)"

"Ndamuka. (I got up well)." That was the extent of my Shona, so all other conversation was in English.

"How are you, Sister Ruth?"

In quite broken English, she replied, "I am well. How about you?" Because all the missionaries at Kana were Spanish, they spoke only Spanish around each other, and Sister Ruth never did learn English very well. On the other hand, she was fluent in Shona.

We walked through the small wards to see the few in-patients. Nothing exciting: Monica, a woman with pneumonia, and Sofie with diarrhea, both getting better; two men and one boy with malaria, and one with possible T.B. (tuberculosis). They also had two women in labor who were doing well, so I didn't have to look at them. Two had delivered the previous night, were fine and would walk home that day. All over Rhodesia, nurses were (and still are) the Midwives and did all the deliveries. Sister Ruth was a nurse and ran the clinic with three African "medical assistants"—women who had three years at a mission hospital training school. They were amazingly well educated, with excellent practical knowledge. Since Sister Ruth spoke little English, most of my conversation was with the medical assistants, and they interpreted between Sister and me. (It was also confusing to me because in the British system of health care, *all* Registered Nurses (RN's) are called "Sister." So just because someone would say "Sister Tendai says. . ." it did not necessarily follow that Sister Tendai was a Nun; in fact, most of the time she was not.)

As we walked to the outpatient clinic, it looked like everyone in Gokwe District wanted to see the doctor that day. A line was stretching around the building, with men, women, and children patiently waiting to see the Chiremba (doctor). I sat in a small room not much larger than a closet, with a small desk and exam table, one dirty window with no curtain, and plenty of flies. I always brought my own instruments because the ones at the clinics were ancient. The blood pressure machine barely worked and the stethoscopes were terrible. It was like using instruments from forty years ago. A medical assistant interpreter accompanied me.

Sitting outside the door was a clerk who checked each patient into the outpatient log before they saw me. *If* they had the fee, they would pay one shilling (fifteen cents) for seeing the doctor. I sat at the desk, trying to determine what was wrong with each patient. The first patient handed me a piece of cardboard the size of a small notebook. This was the typical patient medical record, and the patient kept it. Nothing except an entry in the log-book was kept by the clinic.

"What's his problem?"

Nurse Patricia (medical assistant) told me, "He has abdominal pain."

"Show me where." The patient pointed to a spot in his upper abdomen. I had him lay on the exam table so I could palpate his abdomen.

"Does it hurt when he takes a deep breath?"

The nurse asked him and the man gave a long answer. The nurse turned to me and said, "No."

She not only interpreted from Shona to English, she interpreted in a way she thought would please me. I explained to Patricia—and other interpreters—that I wanted to hear everything the patient said. She replied, "When the pain first started, it did hurt when he took a deep breath, but it doesn't now."

"Does he have diarrhea?"

Short answer this time: "No."

"Does he have vomiting?" No. "Has he had this kind of pain before?" Yes. "Does he drink a lot of beer?" Yes. "Was he drinking beer the past few days?" Yes. Exam showed moderate tenderness in the upper abdomen. Diagnosis: alcoholic gastritis. Treatment: stop the beer; liquid antacid for three days; return if not better.

*

I would see innumerable patients like this in the next five years. Drinking homemade beer was a favorite pastime, especially for the men. They would have their wife—or wives since polygamy was legal and com-mon—make a big batch of homebrew in a 55 gallon iron drum, let it "mature" for two or three days, and then invite all the men from nearby villages to come for a beer drink, charging them each one shilling for the day. (So for the same price as seeing the doctor a man could drink homebrew all day.) I had a drink of that beer and it takes a bit of fortitude to get it past your eyes and nose. It's filled with pieces of grain and who knows what else—maybe insects or any kind of debris that might have been in the bottom of the drum? It had a musty and yet alcoholic odor, and tasted like a very bitter something or other that's difficult to describe. It certainly wasn't like any other beer I've ever had before or since.

Selling the beer gave the host enough money to go to other beer drinks for the next few weeks, and so it went—around and around, with the same few shillings changing hands again and again. During the planting, weeding, and harvest seasons, the men worked hard—right alongside the women— but then during the dry season they sat around drinking beer and talking and drinking beer and talking and drinking beer and talking—all while the women were fetching water from a stream two or more miles away, washing clothes in the stream, getting firewood, doing the cooking, and the hundred other things that women had to do as part of their daily work. All over the world, but especially in rural Africa, "A woman's work is never done."

*

The next man had a "personal problem" and didn't want the nurse in the exam room. I asked her to leave, and he showed me a huge ulcer on his penis. After he dressed, I asked the nurse back in to get his story: He worked in Salisbury at a factory, but was home on vacation visiting his wife and family who lived near the clinic. Since he was away from his wife for most of the year, he frequently visited a "girlfriend". Now he most likely had syphilis and would be sharing it with his wife. I wasn't able to do any tests for syphilis, but was quite certain of the diagnosis so I told him both he and his wife *must* be treated. *If* they were both treated, they would be cured and not progress to secondary or tertiary syphilis. Venereal diseases were rampant among men working in the cities, and every time they came home on vacation, we saw a huge increase in gonorrhea, syphilis, venereal warts, and other venereal diseases. Most companies gave their employees a long vacation for both Easter and Christmas, so we saw many new cases of V.D. every holiday season. "Merry Christmas, dear, look what I brought you for Christmas!"

Before he left, I insisted I had to have both Nurse Patricia and Sister Ruth look at the sore so they knew what to do. I thought they probably knew the correct diagnosis and treatment, but I was there to try to educate them and needed to use every opportunity I could. Reluctantly he agreed, and I had Patricia bring Sister to the office.

Having the man show us the sore, I asked, "Do you know what that is?"

"A venereal disease," said Patricia.

"Yes, but which one?"

"Maybe syphilis?"

"Yes. What's the treatment?"

"Long acting penicillin for both him and his wife."

"Excellent." Sister Ruth also seemed to understand, and nodded her head in agreement. She didn't look too happy at being called away from whatever it was she had been doing, and quickly went away. *Sister, it would be so much better if you would stay with me and we saw the patients together.*

Next was a ten-year-old boy who was peeing blood. That was an easy diagnosis. There were parasites in the streams, and most of the young children played and swam in the streams (when there was water), getting the parasite that causes Bilharzia. It bores through the skin and migrates via the blood stream to the bladder wall, where it matures into an adult fluke, causing irritation and bleeding. It was very common, and fortunately had an easy treatment. This boy was a patient that I shouldn't be seeing because Sister Ruth and all the Medical Assistants knew the diagnosis and treatment. It was just one more case of "seeing everyone who wanted to see the doctor today." With Patricia and the boy in tow, I walked to the next building to find Sister Ruth.

With a bit of edge in my voice I said, "Sister Ruth, this boy has Bilharzia and all of you know how to treat it."

She nodded her head in agreement.

"Maybe he shouldn't see me then?"

She shrugged her shoulders as if to say, "So what?" and continued with her work. Oh, well.

Next: Monica was a 35-yr-old woman who had a painful, infected ulcer on her leg. It started as a small wound, and now was full of pus, very red, and had a foul odor. This could result in her losing the leg if it wasn't treated promptly. I used "saltwater dressings" to treat those very dirty and infected ulcers. I instructed the nurses how to use sterile pads soaked with saline solution (saltwater), keeping them very moist, and changing them three or four times a day. With this simple treatment, the ulcer would clean up in just a few days. Hopefully it wouldn't need a skin graft once the infection cleared. Even if it did, the woman probably wouldn't be able to go the 75 miles to the nearest hospital, and would just let it heal slowly, resulting in an ugly scar. Once again, I called Sister Ruth in for the explanation. She rather indifferently stood there nodding her head, acting a bit annoyed about once again being interrupted. *Patience, Dick. Don't get upset. She's just getting used to your visits. It'll get better.*

Next patient; next patient; and next patient. It seemed like everyone wanted to see the doctor, even if they didn't have anything serious to treat. After a few hours, I again tried to tell Sister that she should save the "difficult" patients for me to see so I could use them as teaching cases. Instead, it seemed like each time I came I just saw all the patients who wanted to see the doctor. I'm the one who needed "patience." Maybe the reason was that *if* each patient paid the full shilling to see me, it meant a bit more money for the clinic, and God knows they needed the money.

Still, I tried to include *some* teaching while seeing each patient, but it was a struggle. I thought (I hoped?) that I was accomplishing something, and the staff appreciated our visit every month, although at times I wondered about Sister Ruth. During the next five years I made many flying trips to the clinics, and each time I had misgivings about what I was accomplishing, but also realized that every now and then I would see changes that had come about because of my suggestions. Change is slow in Africa.

By 3:00 PM I had seen the last patient and it was time to head home. I went to the airstrip, checked the plane to make sure everything was okay, took off into the wind, and turned to a heading of East. The good news was I had a good navigation aid at the town of Umvuma, which isn't far from Driefontein. A tall smokestack at a goldmine was easily seen from a long distance. It was fortunate, because thunderstorm clouds were building up along the way. They looked majestic, with their towering columns of fluffy white wool, but I was well aware that inside them were extremely dangerous updrafts and downdrafts that could destroy a small plane. It got very bumpy and the bouncing about reminded me of the start of our trip to Africa.

*

Just five months before, all seven of us (Loretta, Mike, Tom, Doug, Mary, Paul, and I) were on a 727 flying from Chicago to Boston. We were excited because this was the first leg of our trip to Rhodesia and our new life in Africa. We were flying at 32,000 feet, and just as we flew over the Allegheny Mountains, we ran into turbulence. The stewardess came on the intercom and told us to put on our seatbelts. We didn't do it immediately because Loretta was just coming back from the bathroom with two-year-old Mary. Just as she sat down, the airplane suddenly made a violent turn to the right, practically standing on its right wing. Loretta said in a panicky voice, "Oh, we don't have our seatbelts on."

I didn't know why we were in this violent turn. It felt almost like a spin—I was a Navy Flight Surgeon so I knew what a spin felt like—and the thought went through my mind *it won't matter whether we have seatbelts on or not when we hit the ground.* I fully expected to die because this big jet was definitely NOT supposed to be making such a radical movement. We were all leaning severely to our right, and since we didn't have seatbelts on, we had to hang on to the armrests in order not to fall out of our seats. After what seemed like a long time, but was probably only 30 seconds or less, the plane slowly but with much vibration and shaking, returned to level flight. There was total silence in the cabin. Everyone had just been frightened out of their mind. Everyone, that is, except 8-year-old Tom who was sitting across the aisle from me. He loudly said: "Hey Dad, that was fun! When's he going to do that again?" A collective nervous laugh erupted, the tension in the cabin broke, and everyone started talking. The stewardesses had tears in their eyes—they knew how close we had come to a fiery crash.

After a long ten minutes, the Captain came on the intercom and with a very shaky voice said: "This is the Captain. Sorry about that violent turn, but a military jet was in our airspace and I had to take evasive action. I hope all of you are all right. We are now in the Boston area and soon will be landing. Please keep your seatbelts fastened." We must have been within a second or two of a mid-air collision.

I told Loretta about the thought that went through my mind when she commented about not having our seatbelts on, and she replied, "I wasn't afraid because I knew God didn't bring us this far for missionary work to let us die in a plane crash." I wish I had that sort of faith.

After we landed in Boston and got off the plane, there was a mad dash to the restrooms. Maybe there were even a few who needed to change their underwear. There was a lot of chatter by the men standing at the urinals. "My God, was I scared. Was that frightening, or what?" "I thought for sure we were going to die." "I heard the stewardess tell someone we lost 8,000 feet of altitude during that maneuver." "I have never been so glad to get my feet on the ground." "I wonder if I'll ever be able to fly again?" We still had a long trip to Rhodesia ahead of us, so we were going to fly again, and again, and again. Of the many flights we would fly as a family, some of them also were memorable, but none as frightening and unforgettable as that one. "Hey Dad, that was fun. When's he going to do that again?" became a favorite family story.

*

A big bump from turbulence brought me back to reality. The reminiscing caused me to drift lower, so I started looking for my landmarks. O.K., there's the smokestack, with the mission in the distance. Ten minutes later I flew over our house so Loretta would know I was back and would drive to the airstrip to get me. I flew low to check for animals, checked the wind sock for direction, and landed.

I enjoy the flying, although I was a bit anxious when I didn't find Kana mission right away this morning. The small outlying clinics remain an enigma: Should I just go each month, do the work they want me to do, and leave—without really making any difference at the clinic except for the patients I see on that one day—or should I bite the bullet and try to make a difference by insisting the Sister-in-charge attend all patients with me so she might learn something new on how to diagnose and treat each case? It's obvious that many of the Sisters don't want to change. I can understand that no one likes to be told they're doing something the wrong way, but if the mission is paying for the expense of our gas, shouldn't I at least make the effort to make those needed changes? I don't want the staff to get upset with me, but I also don't want these visits to become merely "social visits" where I see patients, greet everyone with a smile, have a nice lunch with them, and as they see the plane leave, they can heave a sigh of relief and think, "Now we can get back to what we normally do." I wish I could discuss it with Dr. George, but that's impossible. Well, here I am, safely home and there's Loretta ready to give me a hug and a kiss and bring me back to earth.

TUBERCULOSIS

T.B. or not T.B. That is the question. Consumption be done about it? Of cough, of cough. But it will take a lung, lung time. So the silly ditty went as we were studying T.B. in medical school. Now I was in the middle of hundreds of T.B. cases and there wasn't any silliness. It was beyond serious.

November 1970:

"Mangwanani, Chipo."

"Mangwanani Chiremba."

"Mamuka here?"

"Ndamuka kanama makawao."

"Ndamuka." Sometimes I impatiently started rounds by asking a question, and the person would answer, "Good morning doctor." It quickly put me in my place and reminded me that greetings are culturally important to the African.

The rest of my conversation with Chipo was in English and translated by the nurse. I had been asked to see Chipo in the small operating room because the nurse thought he needed a procedure done. "How are you today, Chipo?"

"Doctor, I'm well; how are you?"

"I'm fine." Even though he said he was well, he was struggling to take a deep breath, and had that look about him that said to me, *"I'm really very ill and might die soon if you don't do something different."* Chipo, a subsistence farmer from near Kana Mission, had terrible T.B. of both lungs. He worked underground in a coal mine for many years, and now had two diseases—T.B. plus silicosis from the coal dust. He had been here for two months, with no improvement. I tapped on his chest and heard a dull "thump" on the right side rather than the hollow drum-like sound I should have heard. When I listened with a stethoscope, there were no breath sounds, and as I now expected, his x-ray showed his right lung to be totally filled with fluid. He was in enough distress that I immediately put a needle into his right lung cavity and drained two quarts of yellow fluid. Fortunately, it wasn't pus. After draining the fluid, his color improved and his breathing was easier. I hoped the anti-T.B. drugs would soon have better effect. The silicosis interfered with the antibiotics getting to the lung tissue and explained the slow response. If he didn't show improvement soon I would have to start him on second line T.B. treatment— Streptomycin shots every day for three months, plus another three to six months on other drugs. It would mean at least another six to nine months in the hospital, and maybe more. A long time to be away from his family.

Chipo said "Ndatdenda" (I thank you) as he walked back to the ward.

There were 350 TB patients at the Driefontein Sanatorium ("the San"). It was only supposed to hold 300, but we were overloaded with newly admitted patients. When planning to construct the San some years before there was no thought of a children's ward, as if there were no childhood TB cases in Rhodesia. Since there were many cases, a pediatric ward was soon added, expanding the bed capacity from 250 to 300. We were exceeding that number, and to make room, pushed beds a bit closer, squeezing more patients into each ward.

I was making rounds with Sister Gualberta, a German Dominican Nun. She was a large woman who spoke with a strong German accent. She had been at the San for many years, and knew more about T.B. and its treatment than I ever would. When I had a problem, I asked, "Sister, what would you advise with this case?" and she would give me good advice.

"Good morning, Sister Gualberta."

"Yah, doctor. How are you doing today? And how iss your family, especially little Mary?" she asked. With four boys it was not easy to remember all their names, but Mary as the only girl stood out.

"I'm fine Sister, and everyone else is fine too. Mary's a bit ill with a cold, but she'll be alright. Let's do rounds, O.K.?"

"Yah, I'm ready if you are."

We walked into the ward where there was a familiar odor. It wasn't the typical "hospital antiseptic" odor, but was the smell of slightly unwashed bodies, a bit of wood smoke, plus an underlying odor typical of very ill T.B. patients. It was not an odor that stuck in your nose like that of a skunk, but still it was something that would bring back memories of "The San" whenever I would smell it. Sometimes there was an odor wafting into the ward from the toilets, but the fastidious German Nuns did an excellent job of keeping the facility clean, so bad odors were minimal. Also, being in a semi-tropical climate meant the doors and windows were open most of the time, with a cool breeze wafting through the ward.

I took care of the two large male wards, each having 75 to 80 patients. As we stepped into the first ward, there were two long rows of white hospital beds that seemed to extend forever into the distance. Forty beds per side, each with a small metal bedside stand. There was little privacy. Imagine a huge military barracks with the recruits standing at attention as the Sergeant makes his inspection. Instead of recruits, we had sick patients, many so ill they couldn't stand, at least not for long.

As I made my way down one side, there was a patient either sitting or lying on each bed, with his medical record at the foot. Each patient would spend at least six months at the San because the cure of T.B. was slow. We only made "full rounds" on each ward once per month, seeing the most ill patients as often as necessary.

The chart for each patient consisted of a legal-sized cardboard sheet with demographic data on the front, plus a place for the date, medications, and monthly weights. I wrote patient progress notes on the rest of the front and all of the back. One sheet would typically be enough for a six-month stay. What a difference as compared to a typical hospital chart in the U.S., where a chart for a six-month hospital stay would require several three-inch thick charts. On the place for "age" for most patients, there would be "+/- 60" or "+/- 45", since most had no idea what year they were born. Prior to 1950— when better record keeping was instituted in Rhodesia for all births—there were no birth certificates for anyone born at home, where most of our patients were born.

Now I was standing in front of William, a very old white-haired man and the chart said "102"— not "+/- 100." If he really was 102, that meant he was born in 1868. I didn't think so. Because he worked as a clerk at a mine, he spoke good English, so I asked him, "How do you know you're 102?"

He said, "I was sitting on a bench in the government hospital in Que Que, and a doctor came by and said, *'My goodness but you're an old man. You must be at least 102,'* so that's what I told the clerk when I arrived here." If the doctor said he was 102, he must be 102. He looked a lot closer to 70, but I left it at that. He had gained 25 pounds since admission and soon would be ready for discharge. He would have the honor of being the oldest patient to date at the San, even if the data was wrong.

*

Tuberculosis has been around since antiquity. While reading literature from the Middle Ages to the mid-1900's, one frequently runs into stories of people suffering from "consumption." The term was used because untreated T.B. leads to "consumption" of the entire body. Some people contracted an especially virulent form of the bacteria and died within a few months, so-called "galloping consumption." It occurs in all climates, from the coldest of Siberia to the hottest on the equator, and affects people of all social classes.

Although lung T.B. is the most common, it can affect any part of the body, from the brain to eyes to bones to kidney, liver, intestines, and skin. It wasn't until the early 1900's that doctors recognized that it was a communicable disease and was spread by droplets in the air from coughing. Prior to that discovery, terminally ill T.B. patients typically were sent home from a sanatorium to die at home—just at the time when they were the most infective. It was not uncommon for multiple members of the same family to die from T.B. for just that reason.

During medical school, we had to take Nebraska State Board Examinations at the end of our second year and again at the end of our fourth year. They were written exams (I pity the poor person who had to grade mine, because I've always been known to have the worst handwriting.) One of our professors, Dr. Levine, gave us advice on taking the exams. In a high-pitched voice he exhorted us to, "Write anything. They just want volume. If you can't think of anything to write, write a letter to your grandmother!" One of the questions was "Discuss T.B." I didn't need to write a letter; I knew a lot about T.B., or at least thought I did until I arrived at Driefontein and walked into a ward full of T.B. patients.

In the 1950's, effective antibiotics for treatment became available. Due to the cost of drugs and long-term hospitalizations, most third-world countries could not afford the treatment. Rhodesia was unique in sub-Saharan Africa in having an effective program.

The majority of patients did exceptionally well in the San. They were treated with a combination of three drugs to prevent the emergence of resistance. More importantly, there was a plentiful supply of good food. Many arrived in an emaciated state because of the severity of their disease. The combination of T.B. drugs and good food resulted in rapid, dramatic weight gain, with some gaining as much as 40 to 50 pounds. The patients enjoyed their stay because of the good food, but also because they didn't have to do any work other than a bit of help in cleaning the wards and surrounding grounds. For both the men and the women it was a time of relaxation, sitting around and talking and laughing and talking and laughing. On the other hand, the day of discharge was a time of great celebration because it meant they were quite well and were going home to see their family. Even though they were well treated at the San, they were happy to return to their traditional rural home where they lived in a round hut built with mud bricks and a grass-thatched roof, no running water, no electricity, no heat during the cold season, and a toilet that was either the bush or if they were lucky, a pit toilet—a small cement slab over a pit, with a hole in the middle to squat over.

Rural life was a difficult and yet simple. There seemed to be more joy and happiness in the rural African people than in those of us who have all the things that we call "absolute necessities"—like running water, indoor plumbing, electricity, and refrigeration. Need I mention furnaces and air-conditioning? I was amazed at how generally happy they appeared to be. It was so easy to get a big smile or a loud laugh, even from those who were the most ill. The children at the San behaved like children everywhere, running and screaming and shouting at each other, and finding joy with the simplest of toys. We would do well to be so happy and thankful for the many blessings we have.

Speaking of children running about, we had to warn three-year-old Mary to *not* go down to the San to play with the children. She rode her trike everywhere, and one day Loretta found her heading for the San.

"Mary, where are you going?"

"I want to play with the children over there," she said, pointing to the play area at the San.

"Mary, I know you would like to play with them, and it sure looks like they're having fun, but they're sick with T.B., and if you play with them, you might get it too."

"No, I won't get T.B."

"You might, so you just can't go there. Now come home. You can help me bake some cookies." With that she was distracted, but we still had to keep an eye on her—the temptation to play with other children her age was just too great.

*

Jeremiah was the next patient. Many of the patients had biblical names, the effect of the many Christian missions throughout the rural areas of Rhodesia. Missionaries arrived with the earliest trekkers from South Africa in the early 1900's, and gradually developed missions with churches, schools and clinics in the most rural areas. Virtually all of the medical care in rural Rhodesia, where 90 percent of the black people lived, was provided by mission clinics and hospitals. Jeremiah had a chest tube in place to drain pus from his left chest cavity. Like any abscess, the pus had to be drained or the lung would not heal. It was going to be a long, slow process. He most likely would be here a total of nine or ten months before he was well enough to go home.

"Mangwanani, Jeremiah." Etc., etc. to complete my greeting. "How are you today?"

"I'm getting better Chiremba. When can I go home?"

"Maybe in two months, but you have to have that tube out of your chest before you can go."

"Ndatenda, Chiremba."

And on and on it went, as I slowly worked my way down the aisle to see each of the 80 patients on the ward. Most had very similar x-rays, similar symptoms, and depending on how long they had been there, were either much better or still very ill. By seeing them only once a month it was easy for me to see how each one was progressing—or not progressing.

Next was Moses—*really*. I looked at his x-ray and it was even worse than most. He had three huge cavities in his right lung and one in his left. He remained sputum positive even though he had been on treatment for six weeks. Treatment usually converted a patient from "sputum positive" to "sputum negative" in just a few weeks. Being negative meant they were much less infective. As I looked at his x-ray, it reminded me that I was working with many patients who were infective, and there was always the risk that I would get T.B.. To check on this, twice a year I had a T.B. skin test. *IF* it turned positive, then I would get a chest x-ray. If that was O.K.—indicating I *didn't* have active T. B.—then I would need to take a drug for one year to prevent activation of the T.B. germs in my body. So far it had stayed negative, but it turned positive two years later so I took the drug for a year without complications.

"How are you today Moses?"

"I'm feeling much better, Doctor,"

Moses had gained 10 pounds in a month and did look a bit better. I just hoped his sputum would turn negative in the next month.

I had learned a lot about T.B. and its treatment in my first few months. I saw a few T.B. cases during medical school, none during my five years in the Navy, and only a couple during my residency. Now I saw more cases in a month than most doctors in the U.S. would see in a lifetime

As I turned to the next patient, I heard a familiar voice, "Hello, Dick. How're you doing?"

*

My mentor—besides Sr. Gualberta—in teaching me about T.B. was here to help with rounds. Dr. Tony Davies was the "T. B. Officer" for the Midlands Province, which had a population of one million, 95 percent being very poor black people. He came to the San once or twice a month to make rounds with us on a large number of patients. He looked on all of them as "his people," since he would be following them after they were discharged. Each patient was supposed to take two oral drugs after discharge for a period of 12 months, meaning they had a total of 18 months treatment. *If* they followed the program, a very high percentage would be completely healed and remain disease free. Tony's goal was to dramatically reduce the incidence of T.B. throughout Rhodesia.

Over the months we had become good friends. We visited his family in Gwelo, and they came to Driefontein—Tony, Deirdre, Grandma, and six kids. With our five, it was quite a gathering. Several of their kids were the same ages as ours, so the boys quickly became close friends. The older Davies boys had been coming to visit their "Yankee missionary friends" at Driefontein for many years because Mission Doctors Association in L.A. had been sending doctors and their families for more than 15 years. The Davies boys knew all the "good places" to visit on the mission—where they could get cookies and fresh milk from the Sisters; where they could watch someone butchering a cow; where there was a good tree to climb; where to go hiking and exploring. Mike and Tom were in heaven when they came, and they would wander off without parental supervision. We felt comfortable with them being gone for hours at a time, providing they listened for the church bell ringing the Angelus at noon and 6:00 P.M., running home to be in time for lunch and supper. I'm sure there were things they did that we wouldn't want to hear about, but then that's what growing up is all about, isn't it? When they came back, they usually would be talking about all the fun they had, but sometimes they were very secretive and quiet, with little grins and winks as we asked them what they had been doing. When they were the most quiet was when we knew we should keep our ears open for any "unusual happenings" on the mission.

From Tony I learned that all over the developing world T.B. was one of the biggest killers. Underground mines were perfect laboratories for growing and spreading the T.B. germs. The men worked in close underground spaces for eight to ten hours a day, and then slept in crowded quarters. One highly infective person could spread his T.B. germs to many fellow workers. Most mines did a poor job of screening workers to find the disease early. Only when the man was finally too ill to work would they send him to the nearest hospital for a chest x-ray and medical evaluation. We saw many cases of far advanced T.B. from the mines. On our patients, x-ray after x-ray showed multiple cavities in the lungs, all of them filled with millions of T.B. bacteria.

Still, Tony Davies and people like him throughout Rhodesia were making great strides in decreasing the incidence of new cases. They were working with the mines to institute new policies to get regular x-rays, and to more closely monitor the health of their workers. Such a simple thing as taking a monthly weight on each worker would raise suspicion that all was not well if the man was losing weight. After all, it's expensive to train new workers to work underground, so it's to the mine owner's benefit to keep his workers healthy. Also, the excellent in-patient care the patients got at hospitals like ours, plus the meticulous follow-up of each one of them for at least a full year after discharge, resulted in a decrease in the spread of the disease. It was a long slow progress, and as I would find out in my "preventive medicine programs," progress was measured in years, not in months.

*

"Hi, Tony. Good to see you."

"How are all the Stoughton's?"

"Oh, we're quite well. Slowly learning what this missionary life is all about. Are you going to help me with rounds?"

"Indeed. That's what I'm here for. Let's get on with it."

We moved along, seeing patient after patient, looking at x-rays, listening to chests, observing weight gain, seeing how the patient looked, making decisions on whether to change treatment or continue "as is." Maybe this patient was ready for discharge? Tony's clerk kept track of all the patients, and would get the information needed for follow-up. Each time Tony came, I learned more about T.B. and its treatment. Just having another doctor I could discuss cases with was a joy. And every time he came I realized how unfortunate it was that George and I couldn't have such an easy relationship.

We were nearly finished with rounds, but the patients' noon meal was ready, so we needed to come back after their lunch. "Let's go and see what they're eating," said Tony. We walked into the kitchen, inspecting the three large electric metal cooking pots. Each pot was filled with 50 pounds of sadza—the staple food of most black people in Rhodesia. It was made from cornmeal, and looked very much like stiff rice. I've eaten it many times. It doesn't have much flavor unless some relish or vegetables are added, and then it's "O.K."—Loretta liked it better than I did, and when she had a chance, she preferred it to rice; not me. Each patient was given a heaping amount of sadza on their metal plate, a bit of vegetable and gravy, and if they were lucky, another bit of meat alongside. The patients had the same meal for lunch and supper, 365 days a year. Breakfast was porridge made from the same cornmeal, thinner but topped with milk and sugar. The patients were happy with the food and not at all upset about the lack of variance from day to day. After all, it was better and more regular than what they usually had at home. In fact, when I had surgical patients in the general hospital who were on I.V. fluids and unable to take solids, the first question they would ask was "When can I have sadza?"

We headed for our house for a more traditional lunch of soup and sandwiches with Loretta and the kids. Approaching our house, Mary was, as ever, riding her trike down the sandy road.

"Hi, Mary," called Tony.

Turning to face him, Mary said, "Hi, Doctor Davies," and she ran over to give me a hug and let me carry her into the house. Her initial shyness on the mission had rapidly dissolved; she knew she was "the princess."

As we walked in, Loretta said, "Hi, Tony. Good to see you."

"Great to see you too. How's life in the bush?"

"Better than we expected, but a lot different than we expected too. How's Deirdre, and the kids and grandma?"

"I'm happy to report that we're all fine as a fat tick on a scrappy dog."

"Well, I don't know how that would be, but I hope it means they're well."

"Indeed they are."

During lunch, we heard all the gossip from Gwelo and the rest of the country: What was the latest crackdown the government was putting on the Blacks; were there any danger spots; what was happening with an opposition party against Ian Smith and his party; when would the Davies family come again to spend a weekend with us? Because of our isolation, we were happy to get the news and looked forward to visitors.

"Tony, tell us about your trips to follow-up T.B. patients."

"That's a long story, but here's the short version. I have two Africans who go with me: a driver, who organizes the trip, sets up camp, cooks, and is general handyman; and one clerk who organizes all the files and places we'll be visiting and keeps records of each patient visit. We take a Land Rover packed with food, medicines, charts, tents, and emergency supplies. The first week of the month we go to the Northern half of the province, sleeping at a different area each night, and see between 30 and 40 people a day. We're in the bush for five days and four nights. It's pretty much like camping out for a week. Then we do the same thing in the Southern half during the third week of the month."

"What about the rainy season?"

"Oh, that can be dicey. At times we have to wait for the water to go down so we can get across a river, and it's no picnic sleeping in tents when it's raining hard. Fortunately, most of our rain comes as thunderstorms, sometimes violent, but usually short-lived. Occasionally we've had to postpone a trip due to bad weather."

"Do you see all the T.B. follow-up patients each month?"

"We try to, but of course some miss their appointment or are too late to be seen. Some live in towns and are followed at the local government clinics.

We have men throughout the province who are responsible to see they come for follow-up, and their jobs depend how well they do."

"It sounds like you enjoy it."

"Usually I do. It's good to get away from the office and all the politics going on there, and I enjoy being out in the open. Of course, I don't like being away from the family that much. Occasionally one of the boys comes with me, but they tend to get bored quickly, so they're not so eager to come after the first time. Deirdre came once, and she enjoyed it, but it's hard for her to get away with six kids at home. They're a bit too much for Grandma for more than a day or two. Deirdre wishes I didn't have to go so often, but knows it's important work, so she puts up with it."

With that, it was time to go back to the San and finish rounds. Tony said goodbye to Loretta and the kids and promised to let us know when they could visit again. After finishing the last few patients, I said goodbye, and headed for the other hospital. Tony made arrangements to make rounds on one of the women's wards with Dr. George. Even though he knew of our conflict, he didn't get in the middle of it, which was good for both George and me and for the T.B. patients. He was a good example for me to learn how to stay out of the middle of conflict — *if only* I could.

The issue of Dr. George continues to weigh me down. I try not to let it bother me, but of course, it still does. I consciously try to avoid him at the hospitals and on the mission, but we all go to the same small chapel for Sunday Mass, so it's inevitable that we run into each other. I try my best to be friendly but he just mumbles something and looks the other way. During Mass we say the Lord's prayer: "Our Father, who art in heaven, . . . and forgive us our trespasses, as we forgive those who trespass against us. . ." How I wish I could do that, and how I wish that George could somehow find it in his heart to forgive me for whatever it is that has made him so angry with me. Ah, but true forgiveness doesn't depend on the other person forgiving me; it only requires me to forgive him. I'm going to have to work on that.

Letter from Loretta: *Christmas 1970*

Dear Mom and Dad,

First news item: we are expecting (a girl we hope) around July 20th. I feel the usual tiredness and have several days a week that I really have to push myself to do things. Problem #1 will be how do we get a passport for a new U.S. Citizen? Maybe we'll have to go to the South African Embassy. I hope we get down there anyway before we leave.

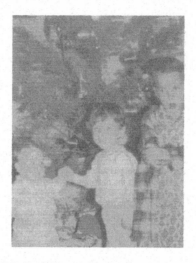

L-R: Paul, Mary & Doug. Christmas 1970

The children got out of school Friday for 5 weeks. Already Mike doesn't know what to do with himself. I will go into Gwelo tomorrow and take the boys, so that will be a little diversion. I hope to leave them with the Davies family while I shop.

Thank you very much for the very nice Christmas check. I'm going to give Mike and Tom the money and let them buy their own gift. We received Paul's package in good shape and I have gifts for Mary and Doug. I'm going to get us a waffle iron and put the rest in our vacation fund.

We had a little excitement here Saturday. Tom was raking the floor of the rabbit cage and stopped to rest on the rake for a few minutes. He happened to look up in the corner of the grass roof and saw a big green snake looking right at him.

Tom ran out of the cage and about that time saw that his white rabbit was out. He and Doug chased it back in, then called Dick. He came with Brother Linus and they killed the snake. It turned out to be another green mamba, highly poisonous. Right now it is on exhibit in our living room in a quart jar filled with a preservative.

Our dog Rex died 4 weeks ago. He got into an insecticide and Dick had to put him to sleep. Last weekend a chest surgeon was here for a conference and mentioned he had a boxer puppy we could have if we could fetch it from Salisbury. One of the priests from Regional House brought her to us. She's very gentle, doesn't roam. Except for piddling all over the floor at night she's a satisfactory dog. Brother Francis, carpenter and bee-keeper, has kittens and is giving us an orange female for Christmas. The population around here (animal and human) is exploding.

It's a warm day and Paul is out splashing in a mud puddle with a pleased look on his face. You can tell he feels he is really accomplishing something. He's changed so much. His hair is bleached blonde and is just long enough to curl around his ears. He follows Doug and Tom around and feels like one of the crowd.

Hope you all have a very happy Christmas. We miss you all very much.

Love and Prayers, Loretta

Rhodesia, September 1970: A huge event for the country was having a West Indies cricket star arrive for a "friendly" match. It's amazing that in a country torn by strife and struggling to survive that a cricket match attracted so much attention, but the native "Rhodies" (white Rhodesians) looked for anything to help them feel as though their country was "normal." In March of 1970, Prime Minister Ian Smith had declared Rhodesia a republic, thus severing the last vestiges of any connection to Britain. Since then, Rhodesia had left the Commonwealth and been subjected to half-hearted international sanctions. During the early years, sanctions had little effect because of the sanction-busting actions of Austria, West Germany, Switzerland, and Australia, but especially the porous border with South Africa. Also, in spite of Britain initiating the sanctions, they continued to provide fuel, and America continued to trade in strategic metals, especially chrome. The Soviet Bloc accounted for more than half of the sanctions-breaking deals. Airlines from throughout most of the world would not fly into and out of Rhodesia, but South Africa Air was happy to accommodate the many travelers to and from the busy country. Any and all air traffic from Rhodesia went first to Johannesburg and from there to the rest of the world.

Sanctions, in fact, seemed to initially embolden the country, as the white population assumed the attitude of "us against the world" and it greatly strengthened the white supremacist Rhodesian Front political party.

Life on the Mission was little affected by all of this, as we were quite self-sufficient in most items of daily living. We also had little contact with the rest of the country, and in actual fact, knew very little about what was going on nationally and internationally. But, behind the scenes, much was happening, especially in the black freedom movement.

MUVONDE HOSPITAL

January 1971: Six months since our arrival in Rhodesia—days upon days of riding my bike to Muvonde Hospital to see the patients on the Women's ward and then to Obstetrics. Always watching the corridor to be sure I wouldn't run into Dr. George. I didn't want to ruin my day by having him grunt at me. *Isn't this crazy? Two medical missionaries working at the same hospital and won't talk with each other? We have arranged our schedules so there's minimal risk of running into each other. We have different days in the operating room, different hours in the outpatient department, and even different days of making rounds at the Sanatorium. How crazy is that? Is it any wonder that countries can't solve such basic issues as border disputes or ideological differences when two apparently dedicated Christian medical men can't come together and decide to work together? What can be the problem? I don't know, and God knows I've tried to find out, but it appears to be unsolvable.* I continued making rounds with an eye on the door.

Muvonde is Shona for "Fig Tree" and the hospital is so named because of a huge fig tree just outside the entrance. It provides shade and shelter for patients and relatives as they sit and talk, the favorite pastime of those waiting for discharge. The hospital consists of a sprawling complex of several cement block and plaster buildings connected by covered walkways. Each building is a separate ward—I have charge of the women's ward and obstetrics. Dr. George takes care of the men and children. We both do whatever surgery is required and that we're comfortable doing. More complicated elective cases get referred to Salisbury, *if* they will go. After my disaster with the rivet I have resisted doing *anything* that I think is risky or beyond my capabilities.

There were 33 women on the ward that day. I worked my way around trying to discharge some of them. Since there were only 30 beds, 3 slept on the floor. Many of the relatives also slept under the beds, so whenever I was called to see a patient during the night, the ward looked like an overcrowded dormitory. Women everywhere, odors of unwashed bodies and flatulence, mutterings and coughs and snores and moans—a cacophony of the sick and dying and the not-so-sick and the nearly-well-enough-to-go-home. At nighttime I would have to carefully step around sleeping relatives like going through a minefield to finally arrive at the bed of the woman I needed to see.

But now it was daytime, the floors were empty of people, the ward had been swept shortly after daybreak, the windows were open and a fresh breeze brought in odors of fresh flowers from the Sisters convent—a welcome change from the nighttime stench. After greeting the nurse in charge, we began seeing patients. First was Gloria, a 45 year old who looked 70. Life is tough on the rural African woman. Hard work, poor nutrition, frequent pregnancies, and tropical and infectious diseases all lead to premature aging. Gloria had amoebic dysentery, but was getting better. The amoeba organism is easily passed from person to person. Because Gloria had such a bad case, she probably spread it to other family members, and when she went home they would likely pass it back to her. Around and around the amoeba go!

"Good morning, Gloria. How are you today?"

With a toothless smile she said, "Good morning doctor. I'm much better. Can I go home?"

I examined her, found her abdomen to be soft and non-tender, and said, "Yes, you can go. *If* anyone in your family has diarrhea, bring them immediately so we can treat them also."

She nodded her head, and started packing her few supplies. The nurse held her back and said, "Wait. You need to be discharged by me and you have to pay your bill before you go. See me when we're finished." Her bill would amount to $2.00 for four days in the hospital. Even with such a little amount, it was unlikely she would have enough. Some patients would "work off" their bill by weeding the hospital garden.

Next was Sarah, age 30, who had pneumonia. When she was admitted, I thought she probably had T.B., but her chest x-ray didn't look like it, and her sputum was negative. Her temperature was 105 degrees on admission, but after two days of I.V. penicillin, it was normal and she looked 100% better. She also wanted to go home, but I thought she needed another two days of penicillin and then I could safely send her home on oral antibiotics.

Lovemore, age 24, was in the next bed. She was admitted three days before with cerebral malaria. Because Driefontein was at 5,000 feet elevation, there was no endemic malaria in the area, but Lovemore had been visiting a relative in the southern part of the country, and as soon as she arrived back at Driefontein she became severely ill with high fever and headache, and soon was unconscious. Since we see so little malaria, I initially thought she had meningitis, but her spinal fluid was normal and a malaria smear showed the parasites. I.V. quinine had a dramatic effect, and by the next morning her temperature was near normal and she was starting to respond. Now her temperature was normal and she was sitting in bed with a smile on her face.

"How are you today, Lovemore?"

"I'm fine doctor. Can I go?"

"Let me get a blood count to be sure you're not anemic. If that's alright, you can go. Check with the nurse later this morning."

"Thank you doctor."

Next was Judy, a 13-year-old with rheumatic heart disease and heart failure. Acute rheumatic fever was still quite common in Rhodesia, and the after-effects of valvular heart disease was a frequent result. She really needed a new heart valve, but not in Rhodesia, so there wasn't much I could do except treat the heart failure and hope to give her a few more years of life. She wasn't ready for discharge. Still, she was well enough to give me a big smile and playfully twist the sheets around her head, looking like a young Nun. I said, "Are you Sister Judy today?"

"Yes. I want to be."

"You better get well first."

Then another pneumonia; another dysentery, this time from typhoid; a broken arm; a broken leg; an assault case where the husband beat his wife and caused severe contusions and a broken forearm. He was drunk when he did it. Nothing would happen to him, and she would go back to him when she was discharged; next was a woman with a huge fibroid uterus that I scheduled for surgery in two days time; next a woman with a miscarriage that I scheduled for D&C later that morning; next a severe asthma that was better; and so it went. By the end of rounds, I had discharged seven women, making four empty beds available for new admissions. They would probably be filled by the end of the day.

After six months, the medical part seems to be slowly falling into place. Of course, I wish I could discuss problem cases with Dr. George, but that's not going to happen. I frequently consult our well-stocked medical library to research diseases and treatments. Our children love being here, and if I'm reading the tea leaves correctly, so does Loretta. We all wish it were easier to communicate with the rest of our family. Mail from the U.S. is slow in transit (usually three weeks), but when it arrives it brings smiles to all our faces. Loretta has occasional down days—don't we all?—especially now that she's pregnant again. Both she and Mary are certain this one is going to be a sister for Mary. I hope so too, but boy or girl is O.K with me as long as it's healthy. Sr. Agatha is her O.B. midwife, but I'll do the delivery. That will be a new and exciting experience for me, but don't know how Loretta will like it.

Letter from Loretta: *March 15, 1971*

Dear Mom and Dad,

So far March has been very hard on us. Last Sunday, the 7th, I had 7 people invited to dinner in the afternoon. That morning Tom fell out of a tree and broke his arm, a simple fracture of the large bone at the wrist. Dinner was unchangeable because some guests were coming from 50 miles away and we couldn't get hold of them. Fortunately, Tom slept all afternoon. Then Dick decided that since he was already slowed down by his arm, it would be a good time to get his hernia fixed. We've made arrangements with the surgeon in Gwelo for the 22nd. He'll be hospitalized for a week (!!), so I will move in with the Swiss Lay Missionaries and leave the other children at home with the girls. Dick will come in for a few nights and one of the Lay Missionaries here will baby sit.

Saturday morning while preparing to go to Gokomere, Paul climbed onto a chair, tipped it over backwards and smashed the cats' dish. He cut his wrist nicely, missed the tendon and artery, but had to have 7 stitches. It could have been much worse. Dick sewed him up and we left on schedule for our Day of Recollection. Paul was very fussy most of the day, but fell asleep at 3:00 and when he woke up was his usual happy self. We brought Valeria with us to baby sit while we went to conferences, and everything went smoothly.

After lunch on Sunday, conferences were over so we took Chris Jackson, our new Mission Helper from L.A., to the Zimbabwe Ruins, and hiked all over the place. Mary walked the whole time, which is something for her, and Paul did a good bit on his own too. In fact, he didn't think he should be carried at all, but some places were too dangerous to put him down.

Tomorrow Monsignor O'Leary from L.A. will be arriving for a four-day visit to Rhodesia. It'll be nice to see him again. I hope nothing disastrous happens while he's here.

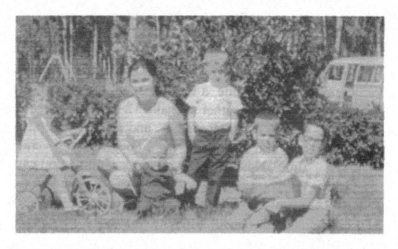

Left to right: Mary, Loretta, Paul, Doug, Tom & Mike, in our front yard at Driefontein

Have you had time to see about the gift from Penney's Catalogue for the children? Tom's birthday is only six weeks away. Did you get my last letter with the check for the flowers for Johanna? How is she doing?

How is everyone at home? I imagine income tax is keeping Dad and Barb pretty busy. Give our love to Grandpa and Grandma S., Babe, Johanna, and all.

Love and Prayers,

Loretta

PARTY TIME

April 1971

"**Y**ou will either shoot the apple off the boys' head, or I will have
you both hanged," shouted Gessler (played by Brother Walter),
an Austrian despot who had control of a Canton in Switzerland, and was
enforcing his strict rules. He had just given an order to William Tell (Brother
John) that he must shoot the apple off his son's head—played by 11 yr-old
Mike. We were at the most dramatic point during our five-hour celebration
of the completion of the dam.

*

Mission life was definitely not "all work and no play." Although I
was busy at the two hospitals, most days I finished by five, and sometimes
sooner. I had more free time than ever, so there was plenty of time to play
as a family. The only evening meetings were classes with a young man who
tried—unsuccessfully—to teach us Shona.

With no television, and not many other activities that took us away
from home, we spent virtually all of our leisure time together. Most evenings
the kids would haul out a game to play: Chutes and Ladders; Monopoly (oh,
not again!); Rummy; Go Fish; Clue; Cribbage; and I taught Mike and Tom
how to play chess. Some evenings we just read, listened to good music, with
popcorn and apples as a treat. We went on hikes and explored. We visited
new friends in towns and other missions. Each weekend, if I wasn't on call, I

would hear, "Where can we go today, Dad?" Or, "Let's go to Gokomere and go swimming. It's a perfect day for it." Or, "Let's go to Lake Kyle to see the wild animals and go fishing." The boys loved to find new places, especially if there were other kids their age that would lead them on exploring adventures.

And, we learned that missionaries just *loved* to party. The hospital day-to-day work was intense due to the many seriously ill and dying patients, so we needed a break now and again. Anything was used as a reason to party: Mardi Gras, ordination of a new priest, a fiftieth birthday, or maybe the start of the rainy season. That day we were celebrating the completion of a new dam between the mission and the neighboring farm. The dam created a lake five miles long that would provide water for irrigating thirty acres of cropland on each side of the lake, assuring good crops of summer maize and winter wheat, and greatly helping to secure the financial security of the mission. A dam-building crew had been working on it for most of the previous year, and now that it was finished, it was a great time for a humungous celebration.

I know building the dam was not nearly of the same scope, but because nearly everything was done by brute labor, it reminded me of pyramid building in Egypt. My boys and I would ride our bikes the three miles on the sandy gravel road to watch the progress. Standing on a promontory, we could watch the men go to and fro like so many worker ants, each knowing exactly where to leave his deposit, then returning quickly for another load. We watched as the cement spillway took shape, and then the thousands (millions?) of wheelbarrows full of dirt slowly pushed into place to make a 200-yard earthen wall on either side of the spillway. I once heard someone remark that African men were lazy. It sure looked like hard work to me.

Gazing out over the narrow river that would be dammed, I said, "Look boys, see those trees up there? That's how far the lake will go when it's finished."

"Do you think they'll have a boat so we can go fishing?" asked Mike.

"I think I heard something about that. It'll take a while for there to be many fish though."

Leaving the boys to explore the area near the dam, I stopped to have a word or two (or two hundred) with Tom Goddard, the builder. He was a short, stout, roly-poly red-faced nearly bald 60-year-old Afrikaner (Dutch descendant from South Africa) with a strong accent. At one time he was a "magistrate" or lay judge, but his passion was building dams so the country would have more water for irrigation. Many areas of the country had poor rainfall, and yet the climate was perfect for good crops *if* there was sufficient water. Tom once told me he believed water for irrigation was necessary to make the country self-sufficient in food production, and he hoped to build many of those dams during his lifetime.

Walking down to his campsite, I found him sitting in a canvas chair, having a sundowner—the traditional Rhodesian "end of day drink."

"How's it going today, Tom?"

"Hi doc. It's slow. Too damned slow for me."

"What's the problem?"

"Ah, two of my cement mixers broke down, so I had to take them up to the metal shop to be repaired. I'm lucky to be here. They can fix almost anything at the mission shops. Otherwise, it'd be a two-hour trip to Gwelo, wait there overnight, and then back."

"Are you pretty much on time with your schedule, though?"

"Maybe even a week ahead of schedule. Why don't you sit and have a drink with me?"

"Don't mind if I do."

For each project, he lived in a tent close to where the dam was being built, being the only white person with a crew of 40 black laborers. During the time he was dam building, his wife and sons ran their large farm. He treated his workers well, but also was a hard taskmaster. If someone was slacking off, they didn't do it for long or they were out of a job. Even though he was strict, most of his workers liked him as a boss and had been with him for many years.

Though he was progressive in trying to find ways to improve water supply for the entire country, and particularly in the black areas, he was still very much in favor of the country's racist laws. I once went fishing with him, and at the end of the day we sat around having a beer and discussing the problems facing Rhodesia. I said, "Tom, I can't understand why the white people can't see the writing on the wall, that in the not too distant future there will be a black majority government."

He slammed his fist on the table, and said, "Never, never in my lifetime!"

"Why not?"

"They just can't do it. They'll screw it up for all of us. Never, never, never."

Thinking I better change the topic, I said, "What about education?"

"I see the advantage of that, because without education you can't teach them anything except the most basic jobs, and we need better educated blacks to help the country grow economically."

"What about medical care?"

"Of course it's important. We're commanded in the bible to take care of the sick, feed the hungry, shelter the homeless. But there's nothing that says we have to live and eat and socialize in the same places. I will never agree that there'll be a day when I go into a pub and have to sit next to a black person while I have my drink." It was okay if a black person *served* him the drink, but not for him to be sitting there having a drink with him.

"White rule forever" was the mantra of the majority of white Rhodesians, even though outnumbered twenty to one. They had been brainwashed by the ruling Rhodesian Front political party in the same way that we in America had been about the black's ability to be in positions of responsibility. Still, it seemed to me that when one is outnumbered twenty to one, you would come to the realization that at *some* time, there was going to be a change . . . It was actually on the horizon in 1971, but would be another nine years of guerilla warfare before majority rule became a reality.

*

So, now it was time to party. Planning the party was nearly as much fun as the party itself. All over the mission you would hear talk about how Brother John was writing a play; how the food preparation was going; what the weather was supposed to be like; and who had been invited. Not much different from a big celebration back home. It also required a lot of planning by Loretta, since Tony and Deirdre Davies and their six children plus grandma were staying with us for the weekend. We had wall-to-wall people in our house during the night. All the older children slept on the floor in sleeping bags. Going to the kitchen for a drink of milk during the night meant stepping over a half-dozen kids like so many logs on the floor of the living room. The biggest challenge was how to schedule time in one bathroom for sixteen people.

All week I was getting orders of "Dick, go to the mission and see if you can get a case of orange soda." Or, "Go to the butchery and get some pork chops and some bacon." Or, "See if Brother John has any of those good sausages."

Like any great accomplishment on the mission, the celebration started with a Mass of Gratitude and Thanksgiving at the dam. It was supposed to start at 12:30, but true to "Africa Time," it finally began at 1:30. Bishop Haene and several other priests were the co-celebrants. The Bishop sprinkled Holy Water over the dam wall and incense wafted into the atmosphere. There was great solemnity in giving thanks, praying for plentiful rain to keep the dam full, and favorable weather for crops. We had come to enjoy the difference in the African Masses compared to what we were used to in the U.S. Many of the priests were dressed in colorful African style vestments, and most of the African people had multicolored long dresses and shirts. The sound of drumming and singing and dancing reverberated through the countryside. The Africans sang and danced throughout most of the service, the deep African male voices giving basso effect to the women's singing. Everyone— even most of the white people—were involved with at least the singing, and many joined in the dancing. You haven't heard an African church celebration until you have heard some really old Ambuyas (grandmothers) ululating— high-pitched "yeeyeeyeeyeeyeeyeeyeeyee," in varying pitch. Even thinking about it sends a chill down my spine. The entire Mass *sounded and felt* like a celebration. We learned a few of the common prayers in Shona: "Baba vedu muri kudenga . . ."—*Our Father who art in Heaven. . .*

It was not unusual for a Mass to last three hours, but fortunately this one was over in just under two—of course, it started an hour late. Afterwards, we climbed onto the dirt wall and viewed the handiwork of the dam builders. Water was flowing over the spillway, and the lake extended five miles up-river. Fluffy white clouds dotted the blue sky, and on each side of the lake one could see the results of this first year of irrigation—neatly planted maize fields nearly ready for harvest. Large heron-like birds were swooping low over the lake looking for fish. Some of the invited guests had motorboats that were zooming up and down the lake, leaving rooster tails of spray in their wake. It was difficult to get our boys away from the dam and especially from the boat rides, but we needed to walk the half-mile to "The Rocks" for the serious part of the celebration—The Party.

"The Rocks" was a special place for parties, with enormous granite boulders strewn about as though some giant was playing with his toys. It was a natural amphitheater and a perfect place for rock climbing, exploring, and hide-and-seek games. Some of the boulders were thirty feet high. We heard shouts of "Hey Mike, come up here and look at this;" "Mary, I bet you can't climb up here;" "Ready or not, here I come." Four-year-old Mary tried to be part of the fun, but had trouble keeping up with the older boys, and anyway they didn't want a little sister tagging along and ruining their fun. Instead she found three young African women who were in the Novitiate—studying to be

Nuns—who were happy to play with her because she was such a chatterbox, and they loved to listen to her "Yankee accent."

The delicious odor of meat cooking over a wood fire filled the air. Tables were piled high with food and two men were cooking brats and steaks, with sounds of fat dropping into the fire with resounding "pops." Everyone was starved, so as soon as one batch of meat was cooked, it quickly disappeared onto plates heaped with beans and corn and potato salad and sadza and rice, as more meat was placed on the grills. It reminded me of when I was a youngster and went to some of the farms in our area of Iowa to help with "threshing." All the surrounding farmers would get together at one farm and do all the threshing on that farm in one day. Lunchtime would be a gargantuan meal. The wife at each farm would want to outdo all the others by having the largest and best feast. We didn't have a threshing machine, and we hadn't been out in the field working all morning, but the people were just as hungry and the festive gathering felt the same, and the food disappeared just as quickly.

Since I was on call, I limited myself to one beer as I walked around and talked with people from around the Diocese. There were several from Gwelo, and I was glad to meet them and find out what their work was within the Diocese. I stopped to talk with Brother James, the manager of Mambo Press, a Catholic printing press that printed a weekly Diocesan Newspaper called "Motto"—meaning "fire"—that was a "fire and a thorn" in the side of the ruling political party.

"How you doing, Brother James?"

"Just fine. How about you, doctor?"

"I'm great. Have to be on this beautiful day of celebration. What's new at Mambo Press?"

"Well, just now we're worried the government might shut us down. They don't seem to like the stories we print, but we only report what the Bishops are saying about their racist policies."

"Is it possible they could shut you down?"

"Oh yes. They've temporarily done it in the past, and are always threatening us one way or another. We just print what the Bishops tell us to print, and hope for the best. We're kind of 'living on the edge,' if you know what I mean."

"I think I do."

I circulated and talked with others who worked for the Diocese—social workers, teachers, and some who worked in the Diocesan Office. Most wanted to talk about politics, and the ever-present topic of "more freedom and positions in government for Africans" was at the top of the list. The Catholic Bishops were outspoken against the racist policies of the white minority government, and there was concern about how the government would react against the Bishops. Would they dare to put some of them in jail? Would they shut down the Catholic press? Would they start doing something against the Catholic missions? Plenty of fodder for talk, but of course, no solutions since no one knew what the government would do, except that all agreed it would probably *not* be the right thing. In giving more political power to the Blacks, it seemed the government always "gave too little too late," and there never was a road map towards majority rule by the blacks. Remember the mantra: "Never in my lifetime." There were rumors of guerilla activity near the Northern border, but no one knew for sure since the government kept the information top secret. They wouldn't want people to think the black population was unhappy with the current laws, now would they?

I had to be careful not to talk politics with someone who might get me in trouble, and even could get us expelled from the country. I kept reminding myself that we were there as guests of the country, and our job was to provide medical care and *not* to bring about a political change, no matter what my personal beliefs might be.

As I walked around, I noticed that Dr. George and I seemed to "circle" the gathering so that we didn't run into one another, warily eyeing each other as we circled. I always tried to be polite if I did come face to face with him, asking him how he was doing, and tried to engage in small talk. He usually just grunted and walked away—but not until he gave me what I believed to be "the evil eye." *Am I paranoid, or what?*

*

Finally it was time for the entertainment to begin. Brother John— playwright, actor, pilot, electrician, butcher, baker, and probably could have been candlestick maker *if* it was necessary—had written a couple of plays and would star in both. The audience sat in anticipation and even with some trepidation, because he frequently used his plays to "roast" one or more members of the audience. "Who will it be this time?" we wondered.

I heard Sister Agatha say, "I sure hope he doesn't have anything about me in this play. The last time I felt for sure everyone thought the fool in the play was me." Today we didn't need to worry because no one was targeted.

For the first play, he had secretly borrowed four-year-old Mary's doll. We were certain she wouldn't approve and would raise a fuss, so we gave it to him one night after she was asleep. With all the excitement of the Davies arriving and then getting ready to go to the party, she hadn't missed it. However, as soon as the play began, she *knew* that was her doll and she wasn't happy with how John was treating her precious baby. In the play, John and Brother Walter—actor and head farmer for the mission—were taking care of a small baby. Brother Linus—actor and expert tailor—played John's wife, and was all decked out in a beautiful purple dress with frills and laces, high-heeled shoes, and a huge feathered hat. The time frame was set when the women of Switzerland had just been given the right to vote, so she and a friend were going shopping to celebrate. With some trepidation, she decided to leave the baby home with John and Walter. The two of them had been planning on going to the pub, but realized this was a touchy situation so instead they said, "Sure, we can take care of Joan. No problem. What do you think we are, a couple of schmucks?"

She said, "Do you really want me to answer that? Now listen, there's a pot of spaghetti and meatballs on the stove for the two of you. All you have to do is warm it up a bit. Also, here's a bottle for Joan. I just fed her, so she shouldn't need it for a couple of hours. You do know how to give it to her, don't you?"

John haughtily replied, "Of course I do. Go ahead and don't worry. We'll be alright."

"I'm not worried about you. It's Joan I'm concerned about."

"Oh, we'll do a great job. Don't worry. You go and have a good time shopping." With a worried look on her face, she walked out.

After she left, the two men sat there talking and drinking beer. The baby started to cry, so John picked her up and tried to console her. (The crying was actually coming from behind one of the nearby rocks, being made by one of the young African Nuns, but it sounded like the baby was crying.) Then John smelled something bad.

"Oh, no; don't tell me. A dirty diaper?" He smelled close to the diaper and theatrically held his nose to let us know that was the problem. With much fumbling about, the two of them finally got the diaper changed, but not without first getting lots of baby poop on their hands and clothes.

Walter said, "Oh well, never mind. After all, we're farmers and butchers, so we're used to this sort of thing. Just wipe this shitty stuff off." Laughter erupted from the audience as the men wiped their filthy hands on their pants and carried on. They just threw the dirty diaper in a corner of the room and left it there. After changing the diaper, Joan seemed to be better, so the two of them went back to storytelling and laughing at their own dumb jokes and drinking beer. After they each finished two more beers, throwing the empties in the same place they put the diaper, Joan again became fussy.

John picked her up and tried to feed her with the bottle. It was obvious he didn't have a clue how to do it. He held the bottle wrong; he didn't think anything was coming out of the nipple so he sucked on it and got milk in his mouth, spitted it out and said, "That tastes terrible. No wonder she doesn't want to drink it." He tried to shake the bottle and pour it into Joan's mouth. He tried this and that and nothing seemed to work. As a last resort, he started to throw her high in the air and laugh and laugh, hoping this would distract the baby and get her to stop crying. The baby made summersaults in the air, didn't like it at all, and started to cry even harder. Just then John's wife walked in.

"What are you doing with my baby?" she shouted. Stomping over to take the baby from John, she rocked and cooed and hummed to quiet her, while looking malevolently at the two buffoons. She looked around the room and saw the empty beer bottles plus the dirty diaper on the floor. Still carrying the baby, she angrily walked over to the stove, grabbed the handle of the pan with the spaghetti and meatballs, brought it over to John and dumped the entire contents on his head. "There, take that, and now get out of here and don't come back until you can be civilized." The two men sheepishly walked off the stage, followed by loud clapping and whistling from the appreciative audience.

The actors took their bows and then John ceremoniously presented the doll to Mary. Everyone was watching as she angrily grabbed her doll from John and loudly said, "You can't come into my bedroom anymore," getting the biggest laugh of the night.

As we waited for the second play, I heard people comment about how much they liked the first play, but especially enjoyed Mary's comment to Brother John. They knew that Mary had all the Brothers wrapped around her little finger, and that they would do anything for her.

The next play was about William Tell. The priests and brothers were from Switzerland, so watching the William Tell story was one of their favorites. We had a special interest because of Mike's part in the play. He and Brother John had practiced shooting the apple off his head many times. Mike was more than ready.

As the play started, we heard the boys from Gwelo saying, "That's Mike Stoughton," sounding impressed that their friend was in the play. In the first scene, Tell and his son are walking through the village. Perched high on a pole in the village center is one of Gessler's hats. Gessler (played by Brother Walter) was the Austrian despot in control of that area of Switzerland, and was loudly and pompously shouting, "Everyone must pay homage to me by saluting my hat every time they walk past this pole. Failure to do so will result in prison and even death."

Tell was doing some business in the village and thought it stupid to salute a hat, so he ignored it as he walked past. Soon he and his son found themselves in prison and sentenced to be executed. However, Gessler knew of Tells' expertise with the crossbow, so he decided on a bit of sport. He brought Tell from prison and said to him, "If you can shoot an apple off your son's head from 20 yards, I will let you both go free. Otherwise, you will be put back in prison and tomorrow you both will hang." Gessler knew this to be a very risky shot, and it was likely that instead of going through the apple, the arrow might go through the boy's skull. In his perversity, he would love to see that happen. Tell was reluctant, but realized that if he didn't try it, both of them would be killed. An accurate shot was the only hope. In aside to the audience, he told us that he had an alternative plan: "*If* I should injure my son, I will turn and quickly shoot a second arrow right through Gessler's heart."

There was much preamble to the "main event" of the shooting of the apple, and the tension mounted. Finally, Tell began strutting about and preparing for the shot. Off stage, there was a drum roll. Gessler, in a gaudy soldier's outfit and sitting on a beautiful white and grey dappled horse, was smirking and looking pleased with the drama he had created. He superciliously shouted so everyone could hear: "Come on, get on with it. I want to see if you're really such a good shot with that crossbow." He turned aside and commented to one of his soldiers, "I hope that he misses the apple and hits the boy. I'll bet you two francs he doesn't hit the apple."

Mike, dressed in a peasant boy's garb, appearing appropriately frightened but also demonstrating great faith in his father's ability, was standing against one of the large granite boulders with the apple on his head and his hands behind his back. Tell took the crossbow and took careful aim. More drumroll. The audience was nervous because they couldn't believe that John was really going to shoot an arrow at Mike's head. Only a few of us knew that the arrow would not even be shot, but that a noise would cause enough distraction so the audience didn't realize it. At that instant, Mike would tug at a string that was tied to the apple and pull it behind him to fall to the ground. Right next to it was another apple with an arrow through the center.

Loretta hadn't been told of this arrangement, and she tugged at my sleeve and asked, "Is he really going to do this? What if he misses?" Just then there was a loud noise and John "released" the arrow, the apple fell from Mike's head, he turned to pick it up and proudly showed the audience an apple with the arrow right through the center. Kessler was crestfallen. Tell was beaming. Loretta was relieved, as were many in the audience. Great applause. Later, Loretta told me she really wasn't worried because she knew John would never do anything to endanger Mike.

The partying resumed with more drumming and singing and dancing in the field, and more drinking of beer and soda and brandy. I had switched to soda long before and took the opportunity to talk with the Bishop. He knew we were struggling with the question of "which doctor will be moving to Silveira?" Dr. O'Leary and his family were leaving in a few months and our Mission Doctors Association didn't have a replacement. Someone from Driefontein would have to be the one, and the decision had to be made soon. The Bishop knew about the trouble between Dr. George and me, and that the move was going to be a sacrifice by whoever made the move. For Dr. George it meant they would be even farther from their three children who attended boarding school in Salisbury. From Driefontein it was 130 miles; from Silveira it would be 250 miles—doubling the driving time and meant they wouldn't be able to go as frequently as they had the past year.

For us, it would mean that our children in third grade and above would have to go to a boarding school in Fort Victoria, staying at the school from Monday morning to Friday evening each week. Loretta would also have to home-school the younger ones. That would be a huge change for us, and we weren't sure we were ready for that big a change. On the other hand, *if* we had been assigned to Silveira before we left Los Angeles, we would have accepted boarding school as "that's the way it has to be." After all, that's what the O'Leary's did. Before they arrived in Rhodesia, they knew their school-aged children would be going to boarding school, and it wasn't a big problem for them.

The Bishop asked, "Have you made any decision about Silveira?"

"No, but I'll let you know soon. I realize you need to know within the next month."

"I'll go along with whatever you and Loretta decide. I had a long conversation with Dr. George and he's hard to figure out. I think he'll be mad no matter what decision is made. I'll take the responsibility of telling him about who will be moving to Silveira, and also take whatever blame there might be."

I knew that really put the decision directly onto Loretta and me. We would have to think seriously about it, pray over it, and soon make the decision. I heard that George had commented that he didn't think it should be them having to move, so I guess I really did know how we were going to decide. But—we weren't quite ready to take *that step* just yet.

Our kids were looking like they were ready for bed, and I knew that I was. So was Loretta, since she was in the sixth month of pregnancy with our seventh child, and had more and more trouble getting around. We gathered the Davies family and all of our crew and got ready to head for home. Mary had gotten over being mad at Br. John, and as we left she told him, "You *can* come and visit me, but I still don't want you to come into my bedroom. I'm afraid you'll steal my doll again."

Fortunately we had the VW Combi Van, saving us a long walk. As we left, Tony and Deirdre commented, "What a great party. We had such a good time. Thanks for inviting us for the weekend."

Tired but happy, we climbed into the van and headed for home. We all slept the "sleep of the dead" that night.

Even though I had to avoid Dr. George, I really had a good time. I had a good conversation with Bishop Haene, and Loretta and I will soon make the decision about who moves to Silveira. I have a feeling it's going to be us. Whatever, it will mean that I'll be alone and the stress of bumping into George will be gone. If we move to Silveira, I think I'll enjoy the challenge of a new mission. It almost feels like the excitement we felt just before arriving at Driefontein, before the conflict with George was part of my daily life. Now we can look forward to another chapter in our lives, whatever we decide.

HIS NAME IS JOYFUL

July 15, 1971:

"Don't push. Don't push. I'm trying to give you some Novocain." Loretta shouted, "I have to push!"

She was angry that I hadn't given her more pain medicine, but things went too fast for her to get a hypo. With just the barest amount of Novocain and with one huge push she rather easily delivered—at least it was easy from my perspective—a beautiful baby boy. *Anyway, that's the way I remember it. Loretta remembers it differently: "His shoulders were caught and you had to pull like everything to get them out while I pushed and suffered with no pain meds. It was terrible."*

"What is it?" she asked through clenched teeth. She still was having a lot of pain but needed to know if this was the girl we were all hoping for, or "just another boy."

"It's a lovely boy and he looks great. He's breathing fine, has good color, ten fingers and ten toes, and everything's in the right place. He's perfect. "

"Oh. . ." She really had her heart set on a sister for Mary, but then realized the baby was healthy, and that's all that really mattered. "Let me see him."

I lifted the baby onto her abdomen. The umbilical cord was long enough so she could hold him as I clamped and cut it. In typical newly-delivered-mom response, she said, "Oh, Dick, he's beautiful."

I couldn't have agreed more. Even though I had done many medical procedures "for the first time" during the previous year, a first time of delivering my own son was extra special, sending a shiver up and down my spine. A bit later, it was with great satisfaction, and a certain amount of smugness, that I took the baby back from Loretta and handed him to Sr. Agatha so she could clean up our lustily crying boy and wrap him in a warm blanket.

*

That night, when Loretta went into labor, we were ready. She was a few days past her due-date, and each day people would anxiously ask me, "Did she have the baby yet?" Or they would see her, and say, "No baby yet?" People everywhere are the same, and all wanted to hear about this baby. They knew we had four boys and only one girl, so all hoped this one would be a girl, but we said, "We just pray that she or he is healthy." They knew we really were praying that it would be a healthy girl. Our boys would love to have another sister, but a brother would suit them too. Mary, on the other hand, was sure this would be the little sister she so desperately desired. We called Chris Jackson, a Lay Mission Helper from the U.S., to come and watch the children. Chris, an x-ray technician, arrived at Driefontein several months before, and we soon became close friends. The children were used to her because she sometimes baby-sat for us when we were away for the day or weekend. We called her when Loretta started in labor at 9:00 PM, but it took 30 minutes for her to come and by that time Loretta was having strong and frequent contractions. I helped her into the car and quickly drove the mile to the hospital, barely arriving in time. Sister Agatha was waiting for us—a good thing too—because by the time we got to the delivery room, the baby was ready to come.

*

Sister Agatha cleaned the baby, handed him back to Loretta and then did all the nursing tasks for Loretta that O.B. nurses do so well. As we took her to the private room, Loretta was cooing at the new baby boy and letting him know that having another boy was just fine with her. I sat near her and said, "Wow, that went fast. I wasn't sure we were going to make it. I didn't think I'd be so emotional about delivering one of our own, but it rates up there as one of the best."

"I wish you'd given me more for pain."

"I'm sorry, honey. There just wasn't time. He came too fast. Anyway, it's over now and we have a fine baby."

"Easy for you to say." Looking down at the baby and smiling she said, "Hi, baby boy. How are you? Yes, you were a lot of pain, but it didn't last long and I'm okay now and you're lovely." Then looking back at me, "Oh Dick, the kids are going to be so disappointed."

"The boys will be fine, but Mary will be upset. She'll be okay once she sees this cute little boy. What boy's name did we agree on?"

"Peter Anthony Rufaro, which means joyful in Shona. Sister Agatha suggested it and we both thought it would be nice to have an African name, don't you remember?"

"Ah yes. That's perfect. Guess we'll have to save Elizabeth Ann for the next one." She gave me one of those looks that could kill, and I wisely changed the subject and began talking about our upcoming move to Silveira. She was tired, so I gave her a kiss and headed home.

*

The next morning I took the children to see Mom and the new baby. As we walked down the open-air corridor that led to the private rooms, four-year-old Mary said, "Are you *really* sure it's a boy?"

"Yes, Mary, I'm sure. You know, I'm a doctor and we know how to be sure about those sorts of things."

"Mary, what's the problem? Now we have another brother to play with. Five boys, just enough for our own basketball team," said Tom.

We turned into Loretta's room, where she was sitting up in bed, but without the baby. After hugs and kisses, the kids really wanted to see Peter, so Sister Agatha took Mary to the nursery to get him. Since Mary was so sure this baby was going to be a girl, she had Sister take the diaper off so she could see for herself. When she saw it really was a boy, she said, "Couldn't we trade him for one of the girl babies in here?"

Sister Agatha answered, "No, I don't think that would be a good idea. What would the mother of that other baby think if suddenly her black baby girl became a white baby boy?"

"Oh," she said softly, with a sad look on her face.

By the time they brought Pete to the room, Mary had cheered up, and was already acting like his "big sister." They all wanted to hold him, so he was passed from Mike to Tom to Doug to Mary, and finally to two-year-old Paul, with everyone giving Paul help to be sure he was holding him properly.

"Hold his head up," commanded Mary. "He's too little to hold himself. Don't you know anything about babies?" Already she was the expert. Pete would have no lack of love in this big family, even if he was "only another boy."

With some difficulty, I got them all onto the bed sitting around Loretta who was holding Pete, and took pictures to send to parents and relatives. Then I commented, "So, now there are eight of us to move to Silveira. I guess we're going to need the big truck and the VW Combi Van."

"I want to ride in the truck," said Mike.

"Me too," said Tom.

"Me too," "Me too," "Me too," echoed around the room like a ping-pong ball bouncing off the walls.

"We'll have to wait and see," I told them. "Let's give Mom time to recover from having Pete before we make any big decisions like who'll ride in the truck. We'll have to start packing for the move, and then decide just what day we move, and only at the last minute decide on who rides where."

"Aw Dad," was the universal moan. "We *all* want to ride in the truck."

"Tell me, who's excited about this move?"

Everyone's hand went up. "Why?"

Mike said, "I'm tired of the school in Umvuma. Our Headmaster's mean, and the O'Leary kids told us their Headmaster's really nice. I think we'll like the Boarding School, even if it means staying there from Monday to Friday each week." Rhodesian Headmasters still had the authority to use the cane for punishment, and the Umvuma Headmaster seemed to take a perverse pleasure in using it, so Mike and Tom would be happy to see the last of him.

Mary raised her hand like she was in school. I nodded to her and she piped up, "I really like the Sisters at Silveira. Sister Severina promised I could help in the kitchen."

Tom interrupted, "Mary, who cares about cooking? There's a lot of neat places to explore, and we've explored everything around here."

Doug, "There's a nice sports field where we can play basketball."

Mike, "We climbed a lot of neat rocks and found some caves when we went exploring with the O'Leary's."

It was a relief that they were excited about the upcoming move. With our history of frequently moving, we had all gotten used to looking forward to the novelty and excitement of a new place—wanderlust was in our bloodstream. Once we finally made the decision that we would be the ones to move to Silveira, everything quickly fell into place. Not that it was an easy decision—it required lots of prayers, lots of discussing the pros and cons, more prayers, and we finally came to the conclusion that it would be most fair for all concerned if we were the ones to move. We liked the smallness of Silveira Mission. I was looking forward to being the only doctor at a really busy general hospital, and I had to admit, it would be a relief to be away from Dr. George and not have to tiptoe around the hospital and mission, hoping I wouldn't run into him. I wished that some way we might have made peace with each other, but it didn't happen and I wasn't going to worry about it any longer. I wanted to leave that behind me. Being the only doctor at Silveira would be a big responsibility, but then, that's why we decided to do missionary work in Africa.

"When do you think we'll move?" asked Loretta.

"When would you like to move? The O'Leary's are leaving in mid-August, and we shouldn't leave the hospital without a doctor for very long."

"I think we should do it soon. We made that huge move from Colorado to Los Angeles six weeks after Paul was born, and didn't have the help we have here."

"Okay. Let's plan on early September. That gives you six weeks to recover, just like after Paul's birth. The maintenance people at Silveira will have time to repaint the rooms in the house and get everything ready for us. Maybe I can fly there once before we move to see if there's anything else we might need. They'll probably appreciate a doctor visit after the O'Leary's leave." It sounds callous to think of a 93-bed hospital being without a doctor for one or two or more weeks, but that was the reality all over Africa. The Sisters were competent, used to being without a doctor at times, and could handle most medical problems except for surgical emergencies that could be transported to the nearest hospital that had a doctor. During our 4½ years at Silveira, we took weeklong vacations and even a 2-month "home leave," and the Sisters coped very well. When the war for independence became too violent, there was no doctor at the hospital for five years, and the Sisters still continued to do the best they could to deliver quality health care.

"What are we going to do about a birth certificate?" asked Loretta. Since there wasn't a U.S. Embassy in Rhodesia, we might have to go to Johannesburg, South Africa, to get one.

"I'll get busy on it this week. I'll call the Embassy in Joburg to see what we need to do." (They sent us the appropriate forms, we mailed them back and a few weeks later Peter Anthony Rufaro Stoughton had a valid birth certificate.)

"You know that Pete will never be able to be President of the U.S., don't you?" Loretta said to the kids. She was telling them what we had been told: children born of U.S. citizens in a foreign country cannot be president, *unless* they are diplomats or military living on "U.S. soil" overseas. Since we were neither, poor Pete would not be able to aspire to such a lofty office.

"Oh darn," we all said in mock exasperation.

Loretta looked tired so it was time to leave. "Give Mom and Pete a kiss and we'll let them take a nap."

As we walked out of the room, Mary turned and said, "I like the new baby, Mommy, even if it's not a girl."

Can't even think about George during this happy time. Since we made the decision that we would be going to Silveira, it seems a sense of peace has settled around us. It's a nice feeling.

Letter from Loretta: *August 1971*

Dear Mom and Dad,

Received your card for Mary and the letter. You have been busy this summer.

Dick's folks sent a box with diapers, nighties, those Playtex bottles with disposable liners, and some terry pj's. They were mailed before the baby came, of course, and arrived yesterday. Peter has enough clothes for two babies with all the other gifts from people here.

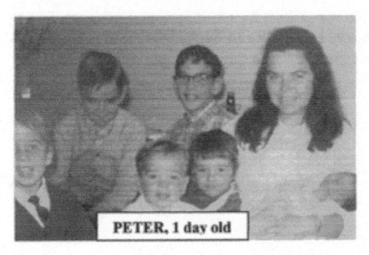

PETER, 1 day old

At the hospital just after Peter is born. Left to right: Doug, Tom, Paul, Mike, Mary, Loretta holding Peter

He's good for 21 hours a day. The three hours he's fussy are usually between 11:00 p.m. and 2 a.m. We've taken lots of slides and will have Dick's folks get pictures made and send them on to you. I wrote the baby announcement ages ago, and don't even remember what I wrote.

School lets out on Aug. 13, and the boys are counting the days. I haven't heard from the new school about what they need, so I will have to call them as I'm doing my monthly shopping next Friday. I told you they will be going to Boarding School, so I'll have to have clothes for

the entire week. I'm taking the whole family for dental appointments and pictures. Should be a fun day. I'm hoping the Davies will volunteer to baby-sit for a few hours.

I'll write a decent letter later, but I've got to get Peter announced to everyone.

Love and prayers, Loretta

MOVE TO SILVEIRA

September 1971:

We were on our way to Silveira. I was driving the VW Van with Loretta, Mike, Paul, and Pete, while Brother John and Brother Walter had Mary, Tom and Doug in the truck that carried our belongings. With difficulty we were able to convince Mike that we really needed him in the Combi to help with the younger kids. Letting the next three go in the lorry meant we separated those who might argue and fight along the way, and besides, being with Br. John meant they would be on their best behavior. I was leaving Driefontein with bittersweet memories: Sweet because of the good friendships we developed; bitter because I hadn't resolved the "problem" with Dr. George. As we drove away from the Mission, I could feel the tension drain from my neck and shoulders. I started to roll my neck and flex my shoulders and arms, and Loretta asked, "Do you have a stiff neck?"

"No, I was just feeling the tension seeping away. I know the situation with George was affecting me, but now that it's behind us, I can feel the tightness slowly evaporate. I'm so looking forward to being at Silveira."

"Me too. I hope the kids do well at boarding school. It'll be different with them gone from Monday to Friday every week."

"We'll get used to it."

Turning onto the paved road, I followed behind the truck, and said, "How did we get that much stuff in just one year?"

"I know. But with eight of us, things accumulate rapidly." Poking up near the cab of the truck was the Maytag wringer washer we had shipped from the U.S. The Browns had advised us to bring it because otherwise our clothes would be hand-washed and wear out twice as fast. There were also boxes with the fifty pairs of shoes and all the extra clothing we brought, plus last year's Christmas presents, baby clothes, a crib for Pete, and various birthday presents. You don't move a family of eight with just a VW Van.

Of course, leaving Driefontein was an occasion for another party. This time Br. John *did* roast me a bit, but it was all in fun. As usual, the missionaries had a great time—we do know how to party. Peter was baptized at Driefontein, with Sister Agatha and Brother John as Godparents—another reason for a party at our house, but smaller and more sedate. Through the mail, we obtained a birth certificate from the Embassy in South Africa. Darn, we were hoping for a short vacation in JoBurg, but with the move and all we had plenty on our plate.

Two hours later we turned off the main road onto the sandy road towards Silveira, and I wondered how many times I'd drive over that same seven miles in the years to come? Little did I suspect it would be for 4½ years instead of the two years left on our contract with Mission Doctors Association. I let the truck get ahead of us so we wouldn't be eating its dust. September is near the end of the dry season and the countryside was sandy-brown and dirty. *How can anything grow in such poor soil?* Small kids were scampering here and there with the barest of clothing and some with none, goats and chickens shot across the road in front of us, and we passed small villages every mile or two with smiling adults waving as we drove by—*now* it felt like we really were in Africa, right in the midst of the people we would be helping.

As we approached the mission, I stopped to look at the setting: Silveira Mission situated at the base of a small mountain. In the center of the picture, a white church and steeple, looking very much like a New England country church; our new home perched on a granite outcropping above and to the left of the church; in front of it were the rooms for the priests and brothers, and farther in front, the Secondary Boarding School for 300 boys; to the right of the church and up another small hill, the hospital and convents for both the Dominican Sisters and the SJI (African) Sisters; in front of the hospital were accommodations for the student nurses and the girls in the Home Craft School; outside the mission to the East was a large valley situated between two mammoth hills of granite. We would get to know all 200 acres of the mission and much of the surrounding area and come to love every bit of it.

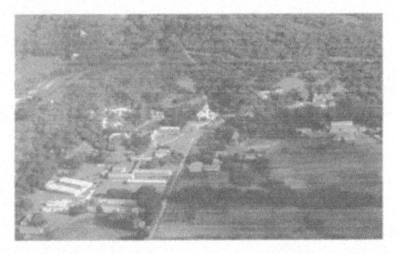

Silveira Mission: Church in the center; hospital to the right, with nursing school housing below. Lower left is the high school & dormitories. Our house is on rocky hill to upper left.

As we approached the mission, a large gathering of people in front of the church were playing drums, shaking rattles, dancing and singing: "We are all happy now, happy now, happy now. We are all happy now, as we welcome you." They sang it over and over as stopped to be greeted by each one. We felt welcomed. Everyone wanted to help, and especially wanted to see the children and learn their names. For me it seemed hopeless to again learn a new staff, especially since I'm the worlds' worst at remembering faces and names.

We were fortunate that Valeria, one of the young women who worked for us as a maid, decided she wanted to move with us to Silveira, so Loretta wouldn't have to train another girl. Valeria was special. *If* she would have had the opportunity, she could probably have done anything she wanted, but the educational opportunity wasn't there for her. She was exceptionally good with the children, and could do any and all of the household chores. On many occasions I saw her with one of our babies wrapped in a towel on her back, standing there with a smile on her face, ironing for hours at a time, humming to herself and keeping the baby contented. She was a jewel, one who made life easier for all of us.

One of the other girls was supposed to be personally watching three-year-old Paul, who had been known to wander off exploring. Towards the end of the afternoon, Loretta asked, "Where's Paul?"

I said, "I don't know. I thought Maria was looking after him. Where is she?"

Maria didn't know where Paul was. She was busy helping with the unpacking and became so involved that she didn't notice Paul was missing. We searched everywhere and couldn't find him.

Loretta was near panic. "We have to find him. Get everyone on the mission looking."

I sent word to the hospital for the student nurses to search everywhere. We had the priests, brothers, Sisters, and mission workers looking. It was getting towards dusk and in Africa darkness descends like a falling curtain, with little twilight. We had to find him soon, or it would be even more difficult to track him down.

Finally, just before dark, one of the student nurses came up the steps with this three-year-old scamp with curly hair and a big grin on his face.

"Daddy, I saw all of the pigs. I wasn't lost," he quickly told me, hoping I wouldn't be angry at him for running away.

I grabbed him from the nurse, gave him a hug and said, "You are a naughty little boy to run away like that, but we are *sooo* glad to see you and to know you're alright." I handed him to Loretta who proceeded to give him lots of hugs and kisses, and let him know that everything was okay. The student nurse found him down by the pigsty watching the mother sow with all of her little piglets.

Finding Maria, I said, "Maria, *if* you are going to work for us, you have to do a better job of watching the children. That is your *first* responsibility. All other work is secondary. Do you understand?"

She shyly replied, "Yes, doctor. I'm so sorry. It won't happen again."

The worry and the searching for Paul added to our exhaustion, so after a quick supper, we all were in bed early. The next morning we heard that a leopard was spotted just outside the Mission gate. *Thank you God for looking after Paul on our first day at our new home.*

And thank you God for this new start. I know that IF we just ask for your help, you will help us through any difficulty, but I have to admit I don't know how much longer I could have tolerated being at Driefontein. Being away from George will be good for both of us, and as time goes along, who knows, we might even become friends. I hope so. Now there will be a new set of problems, not the least of which will be our kids going to a boarding school and Loretta teaching our youngest school-age child at home with a correspondence course, since they can't attend boarding school until grade three. We'll need more help in the house, seeing that Loretta will need to be totally free to homeschool Doug, and later Mary.

Letter from Loretta: *Sept. 17, 1971*

Dear Mom and Dad and Barb and Jim,

We've been at Silveira for two weeks now, and been so busy I can't believe it. We've already had days in the 90's, and it isn't summer yet. Peter is the only one who seems to mind the heat.

Our leaving Driefontein coincided with Father Stocker's birthday—he is the head of the mission—so there was a big celebration. We also celebrated the election of Sister Lydia as Mother General of the African SJl Sisters. She is the first African Mother General, so it was a big day for the church in Rhodesia. There was a dinner at Regional House, and we all sat at the head table. After dinner, Brother John and the "Driefontein Players" had three skits, one for Fr. Stocker, one for Sr. Lydia, and one for us. They were all very funny, sort of poking fun at all of us, but not so that anyone's feelings were hurt.

We left Driefontein the next morning. The large lorry took the big boxes, plus Mary, Doug, and Tom. Our Combi was piled high, with more boxes, Valeria, Paul and Mike and Pete and two cats and a hen too. The cats got out of the box and wet all over the floor they were so scared. We arrived at lunchtime and ate with the Fathers and Brothers. There are three Fathers here and two Brothers: Brother Seraphim is the hospital administrator and Brother Charles runs the farm. He sells everything saleable, and the mission eats what's left over. The missionaries love to make up stories on each other, and about Charles they say that when he was a baby he sucked only one breast and sold the milk from the other. There are four African SJI sisters, and five Dominicans.

The house has only three bedrooms but they're large, a combined living and dining room that's 24 x 16, a large enclosed porch, a kitchen, pantry, small work-room, and a small washroom that's designed for hand washing. It's difficult to use the tubs with the Maytag machine, but we'll manage.

The children just love it here. There is so much more for them to do. We are in very wild, hilly country, with cliffs, big rocks, and caves—all sorts of thing for boys. The Africans are very good to them, and give them rides in their ox carts and let them ride their donkeys. Then there's the cow barn and pigpen and carpentry shop. Mary and Paul like the mission kitchen and sewing room. Mary loves Sr. Severina. She even goes to church with her.

I just realized that I'd better get our Christmas list in, as they should be mailed by midOctober. We have last year's Penney's Catalogue, but I'm sure they will help you at the Catalogue Center. Order them in our name to be sent to your address so that they will send you a catalogue for us.

Love and prayers to all, Loretta

P.S. Here is a joke someone sent to us. I don't know who, but it sounds like it could be from Grandpa Stoughton:

W. C. joke: 1971. MISUNDERSTOOD:

The widow of an Anglican Bishop was advised to take a holiday in France. She wrote to the Principal of a small school in a small village to book her a room. This he did and replied to tell her that everything was in order.

She suddenly remembered that the W. C. (Water Closet = toilet) in these small villages was often far from the house, so she wrote again to the Principal to enquire the distance of the W.C. from the house.

The Principal had never heard the term before, so he went to the local priest for advice. The priest had never heard of the term either, but thought it must stand for "Wesleyan Church". So the widow got the following reply:

93

Dear Madam,

In reply to your letter of enquiry, I have the honor to inform you that the W.C . is situated 7 miles from the lodgings amidst pine trees in beautiful surroundings. It is open on Thursday, Friday, and Saturday only. This is unfortunate for you if you are in the habit of going regularly, but you will be glad to know that an ever increasing number of people take their lunch with them and make a day of it.

As there are many Visitors in summer I advise your Ladyship to go early. The accommodation is good as there are 60 seats, but should you at any time be late, there is plenty of standing room. I should advise your Ladyship to pay a visit on Thursday or Friday, as there is on these days an organ accompaniment. The structure of the building is such that even the most delicate sounds are heard. Hymn sheets are provided at the door. I should be delighted to reserve the best seats for your Ladyship and be present to conduct you myself.

Yours respectfully,

Mr. O. Jones

P.S. My wife and I have not been there for 8 months, and it pains us very much, but it is indeed such a long distance.

DANGEROUS WILD FRUIT

I was in the outpatient department when once again a student nurse ran into my office saying, "Doctor, come quick. Sister Rita needs you in the small operating room."

Entering the O.R., I said, "What do you have Sister?"

"Phillip was climbing a tree for some fruit yesterday and fell, injuring his right side. He's vomiting blood and is in shock, with low blood pressure and rapid pulse."

Phillip, a small, thin twelve-year-old, was lying on his left side and vomiting into a basin that was already filled with bright red blood.

"Did you draw blood to send to the lab?"

"Not yet. He just arrived."

"OK, you continue helping him while I draw blood and get an I.V. started."

With the I.V. running wide open, blood was sent for typing and cross matching for transfusion. We had "walking donors"—students who volunteered to have their blood typed so we could call them in any emergency and they would donate fresh blood. With three hundred secondary school boys, 80 student nurses, and 50 Home Craft students, we had nearly an endless supply of fresh blood. While waiting for the blood, I examined Phillip. He quit vomiting, but was moaning and rolling back and forth. His abdomen was soft, but it was moderately tender in the right upper part, the area over his liver. *I hope he hasn't lacerated his liver. There's no hope for him if he has.* There wasn't any tenderness in the area over the spleen—*I wish the tenderness was in this area, because I could probably remove a ruptured spleen. No one can fix a torn liver. At least, not in this country.*

"Let's put a tube into his stomach to wash out the blood clots. We'll see if that stops the bleeding." Eventually the fluid coming out of the tube was clear. Sister Amoris rapidly rounded up four student nurses as "walking donors," the blood was quickly cross-matched as safe for Phillip, and we gave him two units of fresh blood. His blood pressure became normal, and I admitted him to the male ward with instructions to carefully watch his vital signs and call me if there was any change.

Day two: Phillip was better. He was sitting up in bed, had passed clear urine several times, and was hungry—always a good sign. "Good morning Phillip, how are you today?"

"Good morning, doctor. I'm better than yesterday, but feel weak."

"Well, you lost a lot of blood so I'm not surprised. What were you doing up in that tree?"

"Trying to get some wild fruits. The branch broke and I fell."

"Where do you live?"

"Up the mountain about a mile. My father and older brother brought me here by donkey-cart."

"Are you having any pain today?

"Just a bit right here," and he pointed to the right side of his abdomen. It was soft, but still tender over the area of the liver. His blood count was OK.

Day three: He had several large black stools during the night. His pulse was a bit faster, but otherwise, he didn't look that bad. He was sitting in bed and had a slight smile on his face. I always had the feeling that he just "wanted to please me." And I just wanted to get him better. I hoped the black stool was old blood from the stomach that finally made its way to the colon. However, a repeat blood test showed his hemoglobin had dropped four points, from twelve to eight. He needed more blood. We gave him two more units, and called for more walking donors so there would always be at least four units ready.

Day four: He was again vomiting blood. *Where is it coming from? With a soft abdomen and no other findings, it was a puzzle. Doctors are taught to develop a "differential diagnosis" for such cases, listing the possible causes:*

From the stomach, but why? Did he tear something in the stomach when he fell? Maybe after he fell he went to the N'anga (witchdoctor or traditional healer) and might have been given something that caused the bleeding. He denies he did that.

From his liver? Then it should be going into the abdominal cavity and not into the stomach or bowel.

From his spleen? He doesn't have any tenderness over the left upper abdomen, and again, the blood would be going into the abdomen and not into the bowel.

Is it possible he did tear his liver and the blood is going from the liver down the bile ducts to the intestines? I've never heard of such a case, but theoretically it's possible.

Is the bleeding not related to the fall? Maybe he has something else going on in his stomach or intestines? I doubt that. I think it's due to the fall, but where's the blood coming from?

No tests were available to me to help with the diagnosis. All I could do was give him transfusions when indicated and hope that whatever was causing the bleeding would heal. We had plenty of "walking donors" for fresh blood, but I was hoping I wouldn't have to use any more.

Day Five: Although Phillip looked better, he still was passing some black stool, and we had to give him two more units of blood. I was driving the 250 miles to Salisbury in two days on hospital business, so I said to his father, "I think I should take Phillip to Harare Hospital in Salisbury and have a surgical specialist look at him. I'm afraid he has some injury that I'm not able to treat."

"I don't know. What if he dies there?" Once more, that reluctance to go to a hospital far from home because of the fear they might die there and then their "spirit" would not be able to find its way home and would wander forever far away from home. They would rather take their chances with me, and *if* they died, at least they would be near home.

"Yes, that's a possibility. Still, I think they might be able to help him and I can't."

"Let me think about it." Later that day, he came and reluctantly gave his permission. Early Friday morning we loaded Phillip into the VW Van and drove to Salisbury. I felt it was his only hope to recover, but had the same worries as his father. The trip was uneventful, but interesting to Phillip because he had never been more than ten miles from his home. As he looked out the window, he made small exclamations about the fields, the large trucks we passed, the small towns. This was a big adventure for him, but also a bit scary since he didn't know what to expect at the hospital.

We arrived at Harare Hospital, a well-run institution with highly qualified specialists. Even though there was separation of the races in Rhodesia, the African medical care at Harare was excellent. It was a teaching hospital for the Rhodesian medical students (both white and black), and also for specialist training. I dropped Phillip off at a surgical ward and talked with the doctor in charge, giving him the details, plus a written summary. He assured me they would do everything possible to help Phillip.

"Goodbye, Phillip. I'll see you Monday morning before I go back to Silveira."

With a frown on his face, he replied, "Goodbye, doctor. See you Monday."

With my mind at ease, thinking Phillip was in good hands, Loretta and I had a lovely weekend. We didn't get away by ourselves very often, so this was a real treat. We did some shopping, went to a movie, ate at a nice restaurant, and I visited the Ministry of Health and accomplished all the hospitals' business. Monday morning as we were leaving Salisbury I stopped at Harare Hospital to see how Phillip was doing. I couldn't find him on the ward. Going to the ward clerk, I asked, "Where's Phillip?"

"Oh, he died during the night."

"He died? What did he die of?"

"I heard that he started vomiting large amounts of blood. It wouldn't stop, and he died early this morning."

I walked up and down the ward, still looking for Phillip, hardly believing he was dead. *Why did I bring him here? Only to die so far from his home? Such a nice young boy; too young to die. The relatives will worry that his spirit will never find its way back home. What have I done? For this very reason I've been reluctant to refer patients to Harare Hospital. I shouldn't have brought him here. What else could I have done? He certainly would have died at Silveira, but at least then the relatives would have been able to bury him at home. Mai Wei!* I drove home with a heavy heart.

A few weeks later I received a report in the mail: *An autopsy was done on Phillip, and it revealed he had a large tear in his liver. He was bleeding into the bile ducts and then into the upper intestines. Cause of death: hemorrhage from liver laceration.* There was nothing I could have done. Nothing anyone could have done. If they had operated on Phillip, they would have found the tear, but he still would have died. Phillip was destined to die from his fall—all because he was hungry and wanted to get that wild fruit at the top of the tree.

Silveira brings death experiences on nearly a daily basis. At Driefontein we didn't have the large number of measles or whooping cough or malnutrition cases like we do here in the midst of a large black population. Sure, I had the devastating experience of the boy dying as I tried to remove the rivet from his bronchial tubes. Here I have the experience of child after child dying from preventable diseases while I watch helplessly as they gasp their final breath. How can we do more to prevent these unnecessary deaths? Certainly, not by staying in the hospital and treating them as they arrive. It reminds me of a story: It seems there was a tribe of people who lived on the banks of a large river. They were peaceful, loving, and caring people. One day, someone saw a body floating down the river. They went out in canoes and pulled the body to shore. It was a woman and there was no immediate indication of the cause of her death. Since they were a caring tribe, they lovingly prepared the body for burial, went through the normal ceremony as though it were one of their own, and buried her. Two days later, another body was in the river. This time it was a man. They did the same for him as for the woman. Soon there was a body every day, and sometimes more than one body—women, men, and children. They treated all of them with loving care and buried them with respect. But, they never went up the river to find out why so many dead bodies were floating down stream. Are we like those people? Are we standing at the riverside, pulling bodies from the water, treating them with respect, and sending those who die home to be lovingly buried? We are so busy taking care of sick children that it doesn't seem possible for us to do more. Is that true? Maybe the tribe along the river felt they were too busy lovingly burying the dead to find time to send a delegation up river. Maybe we are just like them, and feel like we are too busy to do more. Maybe we need to "go up-river" and get out into the community and start immunizing children so there won't be so many of them floating downstream—and then we won't be so busy in the hospital taking care of those sick children.

INTERESTING CASES AND EXPERIENCES

Since we were working in "the tropics," it was normal to see the usual tropical diseases: typhoid, malaria (including cerebral), amoebic dysentery, bilharzia (bladder fluke), hookworms and roundworms, leprosy (rare), and T.B. (very common.) Then there were the common medical conditions I was used to treating: pneumonia, gastritis, diabetes, high blood pressure, stroke, heart failure, various cancers, broken bones of all descriptions, and acute surgical emergencies (appendicitis, C-sections, bowel obstructions, bowel perforations, collapsed lungs, fluid in lung cavities etc.) I was busy every day with something new and different—never a dull moment. In our mission classes in Los Angeles we were warned there would be "boring days on the mission." I was still waiting for one. Here are some of the uncommon cases I wouldn't have seen in the U.S.

BARKING DOG

On a quiet Saturday afternoon, we were sitting around the house reading. Our boys wanted me to take them up the mountain for a hike and maybe we would try to climb one of the more difficult steep hills. I needed the exercise, and they needed to burn off some energy since they were pestering all of us. Just as I was getting ready, a nurse was at the door, "Doctor, there's a man with a hippo bite in the operating room."

"A hippo bite?"

"Yes."

"And he's alive?"

"Oh yes, he's alive and quite well, but he has many lacerations."

"OK. I'll be right there. Sorry boys, guess the hike will have to wait 'til tomorrow."

Mike and Tom both asked, "Can we come and watch?"

Since they watched me do a C-section, I felt it would be fine to come and see what a hippo bite looked like, so we all hurried up the hill wondering what we would see.

Edward, a thin short middle-aged wiry black man was lying on the surgical table, with a sheet up to his neck, an I.V. in his right arm. He was alert and talking to Sister Perpetua.

Because we were in the main operating room, we could see out through the clear windows onto the hillside, where several small children were sitting and watching. I thought to myself, *I hope our new building is finished soon so we don't have to put up with people staring at us from the hillside while I do all kinds of operations. At nighttime we couldn't even see them sitting there, so who knows what operations they watched? It's better than T.V.*

"What happened, Sr. Perpetua?"

With a sly smile—because it was a humorous story since Edward seemed to be fine—she told me: "He was working in his garden near Mandadzaka school. His dog was barking furiously at something, and as he looked up, the dog came running towards him with a hippo right behind. When the hippo saw Edward, he changed direction and came directly at him. First it knocked him to the ground and then grabbed him with its mouth. Nearby neighbor men came running, yelled at the hippo and threw stones at it. The hippo dropped Edward and ran back to the pool in the nearby river."

"How long ago was that?"

"About two hours. They put him in a donkey cart, took him to the main road, and finally flagged down a pickup truck to bring him here."

"What's his blood pressure?"

"One hundred over sixty. Pulse is 90."

With Sister Perpetua interpreting, I turned my attention to the patient. "Masikati, Edward."

"Masikati dokotor."

"How are you feeling Edward?"

"Not too bad doctor, considering."

"Are you having much pain?"

"Not that much," he replied, as he lay there calm and relaxed. I thought, *I wouldn't be so calm if just a few hours ago I was in the jaws of a hippo. I'd be frightened out of my gourd.*

"OK, let's see what damage that hippo has done to you." I pulled back the sheet and saw clean, straight, deep incisions down both sides of his abdomen and both upper legs. I don't think I could have made straighter incisions with a scalpel. On the abdomen, I was worried they might go into the abdominal cavity, but after careful inspection, there was no evidence of penetration. The abdomen was soft and he was not in shock, and no indication of a damaged liver or spleen. The two incisions on his legs were on the outer sides and went all the way to the bone. They looked exactly like what happened: something with a very big jaw had chomped down on him and caused long deep cuts. There was amazingly little bleeding, and no evidence of major blood vessel or nerve damage. I was flabbergasted that something as big as a hippo could cause these deep cuts and not cause any serious harm. The bad news was that a hippo bit him. The good news was there wasn't any major damage—just four very long, deep cuts.

At my direction, a nurse gave him morphine. I injected very dilute local anesthetic along the skin edges. We vigorously washed each incision and irrigated with sterile saline. Then we started to sew, and to sew, and to sew. Mike and Tom, although initially mesmerized with the process, soon became bored and asked if they could leave. I showed Sister Perpetua how to close one of the incisions. She worked on one side and I worked on the other. She was talking with Edward in Shona, and they were laughing,

"What did he say?" I asked.

"He told me that when he was in the hippo's mouth, he thought, '*Am I going to die? Why would a hippo want a tough old bony thing like me?*' and at that point the hippo dropped him."

"Yah, he must have been too tough for the hippo to eat. Tell him that," and we all laughed. I later learned that the hippo is the second most dangerous animal in Africa, with crocodiles being first. When out of water, they are faster than you might imagine, easily chasing down a fast runner. Once when I was on a fishing safari with our Bishop, one of the priests was chased by a hippo. Fortunately he was close to a steep bank that he ran up it and the hippo couldn't follow. Otherwise there might have been another hippo story without such a happy ending.

Three hours later the four deep incisions were closed, each with a drain in case there would be any infection, and Edward was on his way to the male ward. With some antibiotics and good wound care, he did fine, and went home after seven days.

Summary: dog barks at hippo; hippo chases dog; dog brings hippo to master; hippo bites master—"Man's best friend?" I don't think so. On the day Edward walked out of the hospital, I said, "Edward, maybe it's time to get rid of that barking dog."

KICK THE BUCKET

I walked into the nurses' station to read the night report. You might think "a large airy room where the nurses hang out" and you would be wrong. It was a small closet-like room with a tiny wooden desk with one drawer, and one rickety chair. A brown-covered exercise book was on the table. Two people made the room overcrowded. Overhead a single bulb was hanging on a long cord from a ceiling badly in need of paint. Whether the light worked I don't know, because I was never in the room when the generator was running. A single metal-framed window opened outward, allowing at least a sense of breeze to cool me as I sat there on that hot, sultry December morning. Flies were bussing around my head. Early morning noises from the hospital came drifting in—a goat bleating, a cow lowing, a rooster crowing, and people of all ages jabbering in Shona. I read student nurse Julia's night report: "Tendai struggled all night, but in spite of excellent nursing care, she kicked the bucket at 0600 hours." I laughed out loud and slapped my hand on the desk. I knew exactly where that came from. A few days previously, I was in surgery getting ready to do a C-section. As I draped the patient, I accidently kicked the small basin that's on wheels. We use it for bloody sponges—it's called a "kick bucket" because with a small kick it easily rolls across the floor. When I accidently kicked it, I said, "Oh no, I kicked the bucket."

Julia was there, and said, "Oh, that's alright doctor. It didn't tip over."

I explained to everyone: "In the U.S., when someone has died, we might rather humorously say, 'Well, old Joe finally kicked the bucket.'" I thought I made it clear that it was a silly saying, and not to be used in a hospital setting. Apparently I needed to be more concise so it wouldn't end up in a permanent written report. Maybe it was too much to ask for someone who grew up in the rural African culture to really appreciate American colloquialisms? I know I didn't understand their culture very well and could easily make a similar mistake—in fact, I once did when I took a medical student to see the N'ganga or witchdoctor (described later.)

I called Julia and said, "Julia, using that term is not very reverent, and we should never use it when actually talking about a patient, and *never* put it in a report. It's disrespectful. I'm sorry I told you that story. I think you misunderstood me. It's just one of the silly things we Americans might say, and you shouldn't take it seriously."

"Sorry, doctor."

ABDOMINAL PREGNANCY

As I made rounds on the O.B. ward, Sister Rita came to me and said, "Come and see this patient with me."

We walked to an exam room where Priscilla, a 35-year-old pregnant woman was lying on the exam table. She didn't appear to be in any distress, but had a worried look on her face. "What's the matter?" I asked Sr. Rita.

"Feel her abdomen."

I gently palpated the swollen abdomen. Instead of feeling the firm feeling of the uterus, I could feel arms and legs of a baby right under the skin. No uterus. Only baby. No heart beat. No motion of the baby. "Is this an abdominal pregnancy?"

"I think so. I don't know what else accounts for these findings."

"Priscilla, when did you last feel your baby move?"

"About a week ago."

"Have you been coming for antenatal visits?"

"No. I planned to come next week, but when the movement stopped, I decided to come today."

"Have you ever seen one of these, Sister Rita?"

"No."

"Well, let's go and look at the book to see what we should do. I'm sure we need to operate and remove the dead baby, but then what?"

We walked to my office to get the book: *Abdominal pregnancy is a type of ectopic pregnancy. It occurs about once in 10,000 pregnancies. Rarely the fetus will survive to near term, when it can be delivered from the abdomen. Do NOT try to remove the placenta. It will be attached to the intestines, and trying to remove it will cause severe bleeding. Just leave it and over time the body will absorb the tissue. Long-term complications can be intestinal obstruction from adhesions caused by the placental tissue.*

Going back, I said to Priscilla, "We need to operate. The baby is not inside the womb, and it appears to be dead. That is why you haven't felt any movement."

With a tear in her eye, she said, "Yes, I worried that he might be dead. That's why I came."

We prepared Priscilla for surgery, first being sure we had several units of blood available. On opening the abdomen, there was a dead but macerated baby boy of about four pounds floating free in the abdominal cavity. He had probably been dead about a week. It was an easy procedure to remove the baby, clamp the cord, carefully look at the rest of the abdomen to be sure nothing else was going on, then leave the placenta in place, and close the abdomen. Not a very satisfying experience.

Priscilla had an uneventful postoperative course. She told me about her husband who worked in Bulawayo, and about the three children at home. She was anxious to get there to take care of them. The oldest, 14-year-old Charity, was with her a week later when she was discharged. As I finished rounds, I saw the two of them slowly walking hand in hand, up the road to the mountain.

HEALTHY ORPHANS?

One day I was walking through the small building we used as an orphanage. We had between fifteen and twenty "orphan" children there at any one time. They weren't really orphans because the father was alive but the mother had died, usually in childbirth. A rural African family was not able to care for an infant. They couldn't afford formula and there was no such thing as a "wet-nurse" in African culture—it was taboo for any woman to nurse another woman's child. We had families bring newborns to us from miles away because orphanages like ours were few and far between.

The father would bring the baby to us: "Please look after Chipo for us. We will pay you, and when she reaches two or three, we will take care her at home." Of course, we seldom were paid, but we had the satisfaction of saving this child whose mother had died, and when the orphan reached three, we hoped he or she would be strong enough to survive at home.

I had decided we should hold a "baby-clinic" at the orphanage and put all the orphans on a "road-to-health" card. With Sister deSpina helping me, we lined up the fifteen orphans—ages six-months to three-years-old—for weighing and measuring. The first two fell below the 3rd percentile for both weight and height. We looked at each other and Sister said, "Can this be possible? They don't look malnourished." We continued: 12 of 15 were malnourished! How could that be? We provided good food three times a day and they should be the healthiest children in the District.

Each student nurse spent a six-week rotation working in the orphanage. Their duties were to feed, bathe, dress, and play with the children, giving them as much love and attention as possible. Apparently the feeding part wasn't so important to the students.

Sister deSpina delved into the situation to get to the bottom of the issue. Being a good detective, she found the culprits: when a student nurse was feeding a child, if the child was distracted or looked like it might be full, the student would finish the food herself. We had well-fed student nurses but malnourished orphans. That was going to change.

Sister called the student nurses to a stand-up assembly and read them the riot act: "Look at these Road-to-Health cards. Most of these orphans are malnourished, and do you know why?"

Silence from the students as they stared at cracks in the cement floor.

"I'll tell you why. Because-you-students-are-eating-their-food. You should be ashamed of yourselves. You get plenty to eat and you know the orphans need the food. From now on, we'll be weighing and measuring the orphans every month, and if we don't see improvement, there are going to be big problems. We might have student nurses dismissed for failing to do their duty."

From that moment on, our orphans were well nourished. Some of them gained 10 to 12 pounds in just three months. It was an important lesson for me to learn: at a large and busy hospital, you still need to pay attention to small things and not assume anything. Another lesson learned: *measuring your results gets results.*

Letter from Loretta: *January 77, 1972*

Dear Mom and Dad,

Received your letter dated Dec 9th just a few days ago. Jeanne told me about your nephew. Mom, I'm so sorry for you both. This has really been a bad season for you. I hope you had a nice Christmas and New Year in spite of all the problems and sorrow.

Thank you for sending gifts and clothing. We especially needed the clothes. We can buy things here, but the quality is so poor. If you can get a Spring and Summer catalogue from Sears or Wards off to me when they come out, I would appreciate it.

We really had a lovely Christmas. We opened our gifts on Christmas Eve. Thank you for the $20. Dick and the children gave me 4 copper mugs. We gave him a Safari Suit, that is a short sleeved cotton jacket and matching shorts. It is considered the same as a jacket and tie in most places. The kids all got a few small things plus one nice gift. Mike got a watch; Tom a battery operated racing car set; Doug a battery operated roller coaster and a soccer ball; Mary a doll high chair, a small cupboard and dishes, and small refrigerator; Paul got a trike; and Peter a walker that he works very well already, and some rubber toys to chew on. Everyone was happy with their presents.

At 11:30 PM, all of the Sisters, Fathers, and Brothers came over and we sang carols until Midnight. Then Father said Mass for us in the sitting room. This is the first time we have had Mass in our home, and it was such a wonderful experience . Mary looked and behaved like a little angel. Doug and Tom were a bit distracting. Tom went out quietly several times, we think to look at his toys in the bedroom. Doug saw this, so at the Consecration he left, not quietly, and began bouncing his ball in the kitchen. Mike, of course, is old enough to behave well and usually does. We had coffee and cookies after Mass. Next day was quiet; we had a nice time just with the family, and in the evening all went down for dinner at the Father's Dining Room.

We had the Davies family from Gwelo for New Years. With their 6 children and Grandma, we were quite a crew. Two boys slept down at the Father's house, and Grandma and Elizabeth Davies stayed at the Mission. We just don't have that much room here. We climbed up Hanyanya Mountain on New Years Day. Grandma and Sara (2 yrs) stayed behind. Tony Davies carried Peter, Dick carried Paul, and I half carried Mary. It's the highest point in the area and on a clear day you can see for miles. We were quite proud of ourselves when the 15 of us reached the top, and exhausted by the time we got back down.

Sunday we went to Mass at Father Verder's out station. It was outside under a big tree. After Mass we hiked into the bush for about 45 minutes to see a cave with bushman paintings . We had a nice lunch at Father's, and said goodbye to the Davies that afternoon.

It's late, so I'll say bye and God bless you.

Love, Loretta

THAT DARNED GINGER CAT

by Loretta

I had just put the three younger children down for their naps, settling into a comfortable chair with Michener's "The Drifters", when I heard a loud crash from the verandah. Immediately a wail came from eleven-year-old Tom, "Mom, Ginger has Hammy, and she's eating him!"

That damned cat! I rarely even thought a word like damned, but this cat had caused me so much grief.

Ginger was one of two kittens given to the children at Christmas time by Brother Walter, the mission farmer at Driefontein.

"Der mudder iss a superb hunter. You vill haf no rat or snake on dis property mit dese animals about," he assured us. We happily received them, as Christmas was going to be a bit scrimpy on our small allowance. Ginger was cute as a kitten and turned out to be a real hunter as she grew older. The problem was that hamsters are rodents. Ginger had already managed to kill two of them. No cage seemed to keep them safe.

Another serious problem was that Ginger considered any meat she found in the kitchen to be her property. Our food was provided by the mission, so once a week we received a large chunk of meat, usually tough beef from an old cow. I had to determine how best to prepare it, and then cut it up to make six or seven meals. Some needed to be frozen to keep it good for the whole week, and that was when Ginger became a menace to our meat supply. In our small kitchen there was no place that was high enough to put the meat as it thawed; our cupboard shelves were all open. With two doors into the kitchen and seven children going in and out, Ginger had no problem with access. If our "fillet of old cow" disappeared, we had a meatless meal.

Occasionally a visitor from Driefontein would bring us some very nice meat from their renowned butchery, and we saved that for special occasions. About a month before Hammy's demise, I had set a small piece of good Driefontein fillet in a place I thought Ginger couldn't reach. My small gas stove had a tiny broiler up over the top of the burners, about where microwaves are placed these days. I put the precious fillet to thaw on top of the broiler. Mistake. I walked into the kitchen to discover the cat eating the last of it. I grabbed her by the scruff of her neck and angrily threw her out the veranda door. She landed on her feet of course.

This is just the last straw you miserable cat. I stomped into the bathroom where we kept medical supplies, and chose a potent tranquilizer. Taking two pills, I pounded them into powder and mashed them up into a small bit of hamburger. Placing the mixture in her cat dish, I watched as she ate every bit of it, even after eating all that steak. *Serves you right, you pig.* I kept an eye on her to see when it would take effect—it wasn't long. She went to sleep under a fruit tree in the back yard. I went to the window to look at her, hoping to see that chest stop rising and falling. *It must be true, cats do have nine lives.* On she slept. Next morning she had dragged herself ten feet away from her previous resting place. Walking out to where she lay, I bent down to look at her. She opened one eye and gave a piteous "meow." Trudging back into the house, I got a small dish of water and placed it near her head. For the rest of that day, as she dragged herself to a new spot, I followed with water—and did the same for the next three days, when she finally woke up and was her old self, but very well rested and hungry.

*

I ran to the veranda and saw the hamster cage in pieces on the floor. Tom was struggling with Ginger to rescue Hammy from her mouth. I knelt down to help, but could see that it was too late. He was barely alive. As I held Hammy's faintly quivering body in my hand, Tom looked at him, sobbing. "Mom, can't we save him?" He knew it wasn't possible but he hoped anyway.

"No Tom, he's too badly hurt and is suffering. We have to put him out of his misery as quickly as possible. I know it's hard, but it's the kindest thing we can do for poor Hammy."

Tom drew in a shaky breath, looked up at me with tears in his eyes and said "I know Mom. How do we do it?"

I didn't know what to do. The only way I could think of to end his life was to drown him. "Tom, I know it's terrible, but we'll have to drown him."

"Alright Mom. I don't want to see it. Will you do it?"

I had planned to ask one of the girls who worked for us to do the nasty job, but I said "Yes, Tom, you go find a small box for us to bury him in. We'll have a funeral for Hammy when the young ones wake up."

While Tom looked for an appropriate casket, I took the quivering hamster into the bathroom. As I held him, my stomach felt queasy. How can I do this? Moms aren't supposed to handle these jobs. After filling the sink with water, I held Hammy under till he stopped moving. It wasn't long. Words can't describe how awful I felt, but I had to pull myself together for Tom' sake. I wrapped poor Hammy in a small towel, soaking up the water in his fur. Then put him back in his cage to dry, hoping he would look better when we buried him.

Tom was being so brave. This was the third hamster that monstrous cat had killed. Putting the hamster cage on the veranda had been our last attempt at keeping him safe. The kitchen window looked out on the veranda and someone was nearly always in the kitchen. I was so angry at that cat, not only for Tom's sake, but for my own as well. At this point he seemed like the cat from Hell.

Tom returned with his box and some flannel from my sewing supplies for us to make a nice little bed for Hammy. "Mom, I'm so mad at that cat. I know she'll never learn to leave my hamsters alone. Can we ask Sister Rita to put her to sleep?"

I had explained to Tom after the second hamster's death that no small pet would be safe with Ginger around. I explained that we could ask Sister Rita to anesthetize the cat if we wanted to have it done. Tom had been too kindhearted to agree to that before now. Unfortunately for the cat, we couldn't give her to an African family because she would eat their baby chicks and raid their kitchens too.

I was pleased to hear Tom was now amenable to having the cat put down. Going to the hospital, I talked to Sister Rita about our decision. Rita was a very down to earth, practical person, and not the least sentimental about animals. She had heard about all of the difficulties the cat caused us, and readily agreed to help. She told us to bring the cat up to the "minor" surgery, and she would be ready for us. I went back home to get the cat.

Tom and I found a large bath towel, rounded up the cat and rolled her into the towel. She struggled mightily when she realized we were wrapping her up. I carried her because she was not going meekly—I didn't think Tom could contain her. We walked together up the hill to meet Sister Rita. Just as we got inside the door to the surgery room, the cat gave one last fierce struggle, meowed loudly and wriggled out of the towel and escaped. Off she went, out the door, down the steps, and into the trees. We thanked Sister Rita. Tom and I walked glumly back home.

When we got home, the children were getting up, so we told the younger children what had happened to Hammy. Mary went outside to pick some flowers for the funeral. Tom and Doug got my garden trowel and went looking for a nice spot for the grave. Our Jacaranda tree was covered in purple blossoms, it seemed a perfect resting place. After all the preparations were made, we gathered under the tree and began our service for Hammy. We sang, "Jesus Loves Me", and each child offered a prayer. Tom's was the last, he ended it with "and please God, forgive Ginger. She was just acting like a cat."

Of course Ginger was home for supper.

BEDA'S MOTORCAR

I was working in the outpatient department when a man was wheeled into my office in a wheelbarrow with a grimace on his face. Beda, a 65 years old short, stocky man, with white hair and a scraggly salt-and-pepper beard, was holding his right leg and moaning.

"What happened?"

"I was coming home from a beer drink last night, stepped in a hole and hurt my leg."

"Where do you come from?"

"I live about four miles on the Bikita road. My son brought me in this wheelbarrow."

His leg was swollen, tense and blue just above the ankle, and extremely tender. As I moved the foot, he screamed in pain. Pulses in the foot were good and the foot was warm, so no evidence of nerve or blood vessel injury. "Take him to get an x-ray." Thirty minutes later he was back in my office with the x-rays—both bones were broken just above the ankle, but were only slightly displaced. Fortunately, the skin was intact, so it was not a "compound fracture," and wouldn't easily become infected. The leg was swollen and tense, but if I was careful in his treatment, the skin would not break down.

"Take him to the small operating room so I can apply a plaster cast." Because of his age, the bones were going to take a long time to heal—probably three to six months, or even longer. We had the usual kind of plaster for casting, but it was expensive, and I had to be careful not to use too much. On the other hand, if I used too little, the cast would quickly break down and have to be replaced. The first one had to go above the knee. After completing it, I split it on both sides and wrapped it with elastic bandages to allow room for swelling inside the cast, so the blood to his foot wouldn't be cut off. It would still keep the fracture site stable. Then I sent him to the ward with instructions to elevate the leg on three pillows and to check the circulation in his toes every hour for 24 hours.

The next day, as I walked into the ward, Beda greeted me with a smile on his face.

"Good morning, Beda. How are you today?"

"Good morning, doctor. I'm much better. Hardly any pain at all. When can I go home?"

"Whoa there Beda. Not so fast. That's a bad break. We have to keep your leg elevated for the swelling to go down. Then we'll teach you how to use crutches. You're going to be here a few weeks."

A bit subdued, he said, "Whatever you say, doctor."

Each time I saw him, he had the same big happy smile on his face. He interacted with all the patients on the ward, and seemed to act like a "Sekuru" (grandfather) to many of them, especially the younger ones. After three weeks, the swelling had gone down and his cast was loose, so I put on a new one. We taught him to use crutches and a week later he was ready to go home.

"Beda, you can go home today. How will you get there?"

"The same way I came. My son will come with the wheelbarrow."

"But it's four miles on a hilly, rocky road, Beda. How will your son manage that?

"He brought me here so he can take me home again. He will stop often to get his breath, but we're in no hurry. We'll make it."

"It's going to take several months for that leg to heal. You have to come every month for a new x-ray and a new cast. Can you do that?"

"Yes, doctor. He'll bring me whenever you say."

The next day, with a lot of helping hands and by using the crutches, he hopped on his good foot down the eight steps from the male ward to the road and then with his sons' help, maneuvered into the wheelbarrow. Sitting there, his white-casted leg projecting like a medieval knight's lance heading into battle, he smiled up at me and said, "Doctor, this is Beda's motorcar." Off they went—the son pushing the wheelbarrow and Beda calling out to friends along the way.

Monthly for the next six months, I watched Beda being wheeled up the road to the hospital, with that same grin on his face. "How's Beda's motorcar working these days?"

"Just great. It takes a while to get here, but no problem. And it doesn't use any gas."

Each visit I got a new x-ray, took off the old dirty, ragged, soft cast and put on a new gleaming white solid one, knowing it would look just the same when he returned. Then his son would again help him into his "motorcar" and wheel him down the road and then up the road towards Bikita and home— white lance protrudinging like a missile pointing down the road. Six months after his discharge, the x-ray showed the bones to be well healed. He had no pain or tenderness. I gently had him stand on the leg. He was a bit unstable at first, but by using the crutches, he gradually got used to not having a cast and was able to slowly walk while stepping on the foot. I told him, "Beda, use the crutches for stability for the next few weeks, then gradually try to walk without them and see how you do."

"OK doctor. Thanks for everything. You did a good job."

"Remember, Beda. No more beer drinks during the night."

"For sure, doctor."

"Come back to see me once more in a month. By then you should be able to walk and won't have to use your motorcar. I think I'll miss seeing it."

As I watched, he slowly walked, putting pressure on his right foot but still using the crutches, got into "Beda's motorcar" by himself, and his son started to push him towards home for the last time. No more white lance sticking out—just a slightly shriveled black leg.

So many people like Beda are filling my days and making them enjoyable. Sure, there are problems, but I wouldn't change this for anything. I only wish more young doctors in the U.S. could experience what we're experiencing—it would result in an avalanche of applications to do missionary work.

February 21, 1972

Dear Mom and Dad,

We have a new addition to our family. His name is "Unky", rhymes with monkey (aren't we original?) He's a sweet little thing, but he bites. He's scheduled for surgery tomorrow—I should say dentistry. His front teeth are going to be filed down so they're not so sharp. Should be a nice anesthesia case. Don't know if I mentioned the kitten we got in January. Puss, the Ginger cat had 2 kittens born dead, and a week later one live one. It is striped ginger and eggshell. Blackie disappeared two weeks ago so we can keep this one as replacement.

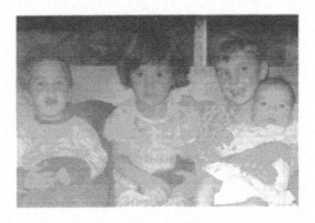

L-R: Paul, Mary, Doug, Peter

We are currently entertaining a nasty cough. One at a time, we seem to be taking turns. I've had it for the last few days. It doesn't sound as bad as it feels. Poor Peter and Paul went through it with hardly an aspirin. I'm getting dosed up good and proper to try to prevent it getting worse.

Sunday we spent the day at Kyle Game reserve, viewing game and fishing and picnicking. It was a beautiful day, and we saw lots of animals, and Dick and the boys caught some bass. When we got home, we found the mission was having a party, the last before Lent. Dick went over to offer our apologies but didn't come home. Well, first thing I knew, Sister Rita came knocking at the door, dressed in a dirndl and peasant blouse and huge flowered hat, and Sister Perpetua dressed like an African Man, with floppy hat, large shirt and baggy pants and fake mustache. They came to invite me to the party, so I quickly got the young ones tucked in and gave Mike instructions for the rest. Everyone was in costume, but I couldn't think of anything, so I came as me. It really was fun. I stayed for an hour and then went back to feed Peter.

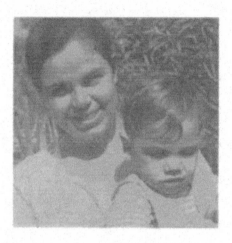

Loretta with Peter

Of course I missed the best. They decided to play a joke on the student nurses, so sister Perpetua and Brother Seraphim got into Father's car and drove up to the hospital. Brother told them he had a very sick man and they must go get the Doctor. They took Sister—the 'sick man'— into the Men's ward, but she refused to allow them to undress her, then refused to give any history, just hugged her stomach and moaned and groaned. One student came to get Dick, and was very embarrassed to see all the Sisters in costumes. She recognized the Dominican Sisters, but didn't realize the African Sisters were in civilian clothes—thought they were just guests. Dick sent the student over to the African convent to get Sister Letetia, because she was on call. She went up and as soon as she saw Sister Perpetua, she knew it was a prank and said they must take this patient to outpatient as he was so difficult and was disturbing all the others. Then she said since he was so uncooperative, that she would take the history and they could go back to work. Then the patient ran away. Sister tried to explain that it was all a joke, but the girls wouldn't believe her. They thought she was saying that so that they wouldn't be frightened. The next morning there were all sorts of stories going around.

Peter is sitting up by himself now and pulls himself up to a kneeling position very easily. Once in a while I hear a desperate cry and find him standing. He really keeps us busy while he is awake. He's lost a lot of his fat since he has been so active. I'm glad. I'm afraid Paul is going to be our fatty. The girls just can't listen to him cry and give him cookies or bread and jelly whenever I'm not standing right over them. Every place we walk on the mission, someone gives them sweets. Don't know why Mary isn't fat cause she gets the same treats. Bye for now. How did you like the W.C. story?

Love and Prayers, Loretta

NYOKA

by Loretta

It was a beautiful spring Sunday on the mission. The jacaranda trees were in full purple bloom and the msasa trees were glowing in their soft coral-pink leaves. Our rains had begun early, so the gloomy concerns about whether we would have a good planting season were past. New green grass was covering what had been dry and bare ground, and people were industriously hoeing their fields.

Each Sunday after Mass the Dominican's had an "open house" for anyone who wanted a nice cup of real German coffee, with perhaps a teaspoon of Schnapps in it. We took the children home for Valeria to look after and then hurried up the hill to the convent. We could hear Vita's excited voice as we neared the convent.

Sister Vita, in her early forties, was one of those people who lived life with great enthusiasm. Her face seemed to glow with joy and she brought a happy energy into any room she entered. She had been assigned to Silveira Hospital temporarily while she waited for things to be arranged for a new mission in Bolivia. The Dominican Sisters were sending her with another Sister so they could establish a base for a new Mission Outreach station. As we approached the open door we heard her say, "What a glorious day. Let's not waste it indoors. We should all go for a walk."

"Marvelous idea, perhaps we can put together a picnic," agreed Sister Rosemary.

"We should go to the Falls. They'll be beautiful after the rain we've had." said Father Verder.

Upon entering the sitting room, we were warmly greeted. There was a large group that day: the Dominican's—Rita, Vita, Rosemary, Amoris, Agatha, and Waltroud; the two out-station priests, the Father Superior of the mission, the two priests from the Secondary School, and two SJI Sisters. It looked as though there would be no place to sit.

"Loretta, come sit with me," invited Vita, as she moved over on the small settee, and someone else found a small stool for Dick.

"What is this we heard about a picnic at the Falls?" I asked.

"We were just saying that the day is calling us out of doors. We want to do something to celebrate this fine weather," said Rosemary.

We quickly organized a picnic. Every group was to provide something. The Bethlehem priests and brothers provided soda and beer, the SJI sisters volunteered brats and rolls, the Dominicans would bring a salad, and I would bring dessert. I had baked a large cake the day before that would be perfect.

The place we called the "Falls" was more like a rapids that flowed steeply downhill over granite boulders for two-hundred yards. The water would really be boiling over those rocks during the rainy season, and the sound of rushing water would feel like a soothing balm after a long, cold and drizzly winter.

We walked the mile and a half together, all happily chattering about events at the hospital and Secondary School. Sister Vita's cheerfulness was infectious. Our three older boys, Mike, Tom, and Doug, along with five-year-old Mary, ran and climbed the boulders and small trees as we ambled along. Dick and the priests took turns carrying Paul on their shoulders, while I had Peter on my back, African style, tied securely with a wrap-around towel.

The area of the Falls was quite hilly, covered with large rocks and slabs of granite that were typical of the Bikita District. There were many msasa and other bush trees to provide shade, as well as various types of aloe plants. The first time we went to the Falls we were stopped in our tracks by the beauty of the scene. It was in the Fall Season and the aloe plants Excelsia were in full bloom—hundreds of them, many over six-feet tall, with six to twelve candelabra branches of fiery red blossoms. We had never seen so many in one place—it made me think of the Garden of Eden. Since it was Spring, the aloes weren't blooming, but the msasa trees were in glorious shades of orange and coral.

Our picnic place was next to the stream with a good view of the falls. At the steepest spot, a large granite ledge acted as a barrier to keep the children from falling over the edge. A flat area twelve by eight feet had shallow depressions here and there that were perfect places for the serving dishes. Vita placed my towel-covered cake in the center of one, the men started a fire to cook the brats, and the rest of us found places to sit. Mary, our little monkey, was climbing all around us when she slipped and quite suddenly sat down. Vita laughed and said, "Mary, you've found a lovely place to sit."

She looked up with a frown on her face and said, "I think I'm sitting on the cake."

Vita picked her up, twirled her around, and sat her on a safe spot. She took the towel off the cake and there was an indentation exactly matching Mary's little bottom. Vita laughingly said, "You certainly were. But don't worry, it isn't spoiled," and gave Mary another hug.

Everyone laughed and assured Mary the cake was all right, so she soon recovered her spirits and was climbing rocks once again with the boys. That afternoon remains as one of my favorite memories: the warm sunny day, the rushing water, the easy camaraderie of our missionary friends, the good food, and the good fellowship. We all were on one side of the river, while down on the rocks on the other side and at the bottom of the falls were three women doing their family laundry. Their children were playing in the stream and running up the hill on the other side, laughing and jabbering in Shona and pointing at all the "murungus"—white people—sitting across from them.

After eating we lazily sat around and visited. Brother Charles was napping under a tree near the edge of the stream when the boys on the other side began shouting, "Nyoka! Nyoka! (snake, snake)," while pointing at the tree above Charles.

"Charles, Charles," Father Verder called. He woke and quickly stood as we all gathered around the tree, trying unsuccessfully to see the snake. We could only see the branches.

"Look, there on the right side of the trunk, half way up. It looks exactly like a small branch sticking straight out, but you can see it's red mouth and a tongue flickering in and out," said Father Verder.

"I see it," said Mike, as he and Tom squeezed past the grownups to get under the tree. Soon we all were able to see it.

"It's a Twig Snake. Doesn't it look like a twig sticking straight out?" said Verder. "It used to be considered harmless, but in recent years the venom of all snakes has been tested, and this one is very poisonous. It's not aggressive, so even when threatened, it rarely bites."

Although snakes are actually helpful to farmers by killing rodents, rarely does anyone—black or white—consider them an ally, so the men quickly dispatched the snake.

After so much food, excitement, and exercise, we were tired and it was time to go home. We packed the leftovers and began the mile-and-a-half trek back to the mission. Dick picked up the snake, wrapped it around his neck like some brave white hunter and said, "I'll take this with me to put it in a jar with preservatives and display it in my office. Patients will love it."

Snakes are always a good topic of conversation, even in Africa where there are so many. We had walked a short distance when the snake suddenly tightened around Dick's neck and began moving. He yelled, desperately flung it off, and Charles proceeded to kill it once again. This time the head was nearly off, so we felt that it surely was dead this time. Still, Dick carried it gingerly at arms length the rest of the way home.

When we arrived home, I put the little ones—Paul, Mary, and Peter—down for a nap, and Dick and I went to our bedroom. A little beer and a long walk meant we were ready for a nice Sunday afternoon siesta.

We were wakened by someone pounding on our porch door, shouting "Dokta, Dokta, come quickly, you're wanted in Maternity." Chrysanthemum, one of our nursing students was there. "Dokta, Dokta, come quickly! You must come soon."

Dick ran to the door and soon was back to announce what I already knew—he had to go for a C-section. I stayed in bed, but heard him speak to Mary as he left the house. "Mary, what are you doing? You know Mommy doesn't want you digging in her flowers."

Oh no, I groaned to myself. *I just planted those flowers yesterday.* Growing a flower border had been a constant battle. I had to defend it from cattle at midnight, from our dog who thought the nice black dirt was great for digging, and from Mary who thought the same as our dog, only she used it for mud pies. I reluctantly got up to see what Mary was doing. There she was, her cute little pink and white shorts-outfit streaked in mud, curly brown hair damp with sweat around her grubby face, her head bent down but eyes looking up at me.

"Mary! You know you aren't supposed to play in my flower garden. I just planted those seedlings yesterday," I said in an exasperated voice. "I'm *so* angry. I could give you a good spanking."

She softly replied, "Mommy, God doesn't want you to be angry. Why don't we *both* just say we're sorry?"

I went from anger to elation in a second. I was home-schooling Mary, and we had just been talking about how God loves us, and how the things we do can make him pleased with us or unhappy. *Yes! She got it.*

"You're right Mary, you go first."

"Okay, I'm sorry for messing up your garden Mommy."

"I forgive you Mary and I love you. I'm sorry I was so angry. Will you forgive me?"

"Yes Mommy."

"Then let's have a big hug and a kiss." I held out my arms as she wrapped her grubby hands and arms tightly around my neck.

"Now Mary, God's happy we've said we're sorry, but we need to do something more. When you hurt someone, you need to try to make it better if you can. Now you need to help fix my flowerbed. Let's see what needs to be done."

We walked to the flowerbed and I said, "First you need to put all the dirt back inside the bed and smooth it out. You pulled three plants out, so I'll replant them after you smooth the dirt. Okay?"

"Okay Mommy. I can do it." It really wasn't that messed up. I was just frustrated at her for getting into it again. We finished in ten minutes, and if I had done it by myself it would have been five.

"You know Mary, I think we can find a good place for you to make your mud pies over by that plumeria tree. Let's go and look." We walked to the edge of the lawn where there was a rock wall with a nice smooth ledge. "Nothing is planted here by the wall, there's a lot of dirt to work with, and the ledge is a good place to put the mud pies so they can dry." *Why didn't I think of this before?* I leaned over, kissed her and said, "Now you need a bath before dinner. Go wake the boys, and then take a bath. I'll go in and start dinner."

"Okay Mommy," and off she scampered.

MEASLES & WHOOPING COUGH

L oud banging on the screen door in the middle of the night: "Doctor, Doctor, come quick. Tendai is gasping." I knew that Tendai was extremely ill with measles, plus swelling of the upper airway. We had her in a "croup tent" with high humidity oxygen—which we really couldn't afford. It was our only hope to save this child. In nearly all such cases, when a student nurse came with the message "Tendai (or whoever) is gasping . . ." it really meant the child was near death, and there was nothing more for me to do. Still, I ran down the hill, around the back of the church, and up the hill to the hospital—all in the dark because the generator wasn't on during the night—to be with the child and mother. I went to let the mother and nurses know I deeply cared about the welfare of every patient, even when there was nothing more I could do to help.

As I breathlessly arrived on the pediatric ward, I used a flashlight to peer into the fog of the mist tent and watched Tendai take her last few breaths and quietly die. She was four years old and weighed only 16 pounds. She had been admitted chronically ill with recurrent diarrhea. As we treated the diarrhea, she contracted measles—that damnable "hospital contact measles."

*

During the measles season we would have ill children on the open ward without realizing they also were incubating the measles virus and spreading it to everyone else. Those on the ward who hadn't previously had measles would be exposed, and many would develop a severe case because of their malnutrition and depressed immunity. The 20 beds on our main pediatric ward were full most of the time, with everyone being exposed to each other's communicable diseases. We couldn't afford smaller isolation rooms and we couldn't afford the vaccine that would have prevented the spread of measles.

The epidemic season lasted from May to October, our winter season. As much as possible we isolated those with measles or whooping cough. When an ill child with some other disease arrived, we preferred to treat them at home, but some were too ill to be sent home, so we nearly always had a full ward. It was terribly discouraging to nurse a child through a bout of typhoid fever, only to have her get "hospital contact measles," and die ten days later. If only we had measles vaccine.

*

Once again I watched as the mother threw herself onto the cement floor, loudly wailing and keening. On and on it went—to me it felt like an hour but was probably only ten minutes—as I stood by helplessly, knowing it didn't make any difference what I said or what I did. The mother had to go through the ritual. Then got up and put the dead child on her back, secured her there with a towel wrapped around them both. Gathering her cooking utensils, food, and clothing, she started for home—even at three AM. As she passed other mothers on the ward, she again started keening so all knew of her sorrow. Even as she left the hospital in the dark, we could hear her cries as she slowly ascended the road up the mountain.

Two nights later, once again pounding on the screen door. "Doctor, Julia is gasping."

Same situation—different cause. Julia, a cute four-year-old, was completely healthy until two weeks before admission. She had a cough that progressively became worse. We finally diagnosed whooping cough and treated her with the appropriate antibiotics, but her upper airway gradually swelled to the point of not allowing air into her lungs. As a last-ditch effort, I did a tracheotomy—an opening into her windpipe—hoping this would improve the airflow. She was placed in the high humidity, high oxygen-content mist tent. When I left the ward the previous evening, she was holding her own and I hoped that IF we kept her alive another day or two, the swelling would go down and she would survive. I was doing all I could—and prayed that it was enough.

It was not. As I reached her cot, I could see she had just died. Same scenario: sadly tell the mother; same grief reaction; same feeling of helplessness; same sad trudge down the hill and up the hill to our house in the dark; same sleepless night as I fretted over the frequent but preventable deaths. In Julia's case, I felt even worse, because we *did* have vaccination against whooping cough, giving it to all who came to our baby-clinics. The problem was, we didn't go very far from the hospital and Julia lived 10 miles away. Such an easy prevention—*an ounce of prevention is worth a pound of cure, but not for Julia.*

My God, my God, why are you abandoning these poor people?

I imagined I might have heard, "I'm not abandoning them. I sent you."

"Oh. But what can I do? How do I solve such a big problem?

"You will find a way."

"Thanks, but I was hoping for directions and a plan. I'm good at following directions. I don't know about dreaming up a plan on my own."

"You won't be on your own."

"Oh."

Two days later, another measles death during the day. Same grief process, but a different story. The child died of upper airway obstruction due to measles, but *not* in the mist-tent. The mother refused to let us put him in there, because she believed there must be an evil spirit in the tent since so many children were dying there. Even though in some cases it was very helpful in relieving upper airway swelling, we were not able to use it at all for two months in order to allow the situation to calm down. Then I used it on less serious cases so the women could see that most of the children recovered.

Watching the mothers go through the gut-wrenching grief was heart-breaking for all of us. But, because we heard it so often, we had become somewhat hardened to it. *Is it truly possible that we get "hardened to the death of a child?" How can that happen? Is this what happens in war? "Oh, it's just another day. We only lost seven men today!" "Oh, it's just another measles and whooping cough season. We only lost 50 this year." How can I continue to come to the hospital day after day to watch children die of preventable diseases? Where is that plan, God?*

*

So far that year, we had 130 children with measles, 25% contracting it after being admitted. Thirty-five died. Twenty-five cases of whooping cough, with five deaths. How can this be? Whooping cough had been eliminated in the rich world by routinely giving DPT vaccine to all children. Most people in the U.S. thought of measles as a "normal childhood disease" with low mortality, but of course that wasn't true. The "developed world" produced measles vaccine because doctors *knew* measles had a small but real mortality rate—even in otherwise healthy children—and definitely a high morbidity rate. Many children were seriously ill during the ten-days of illness, and some of them ended up with life-long health problems. Because of the vaccine, measles had become almost non-existent in the U.S. Not so in Africa. Each year we had a measles epidemic, with a severe one every three to four years. This year it was severe. In Africa there was a saying, "Don't count the number of children you have until they've had *biri-piri*—measles." The local people knew the seriousness of this common childhood disease. I was just praying that God would soon reveal His plan to me.

*

How to vaccinate all children under five years old in a District measuring 20 by 25 miles (500 square miles), with bad sandy roads and no direct communication? Simple, you only need to:

Arrange a meeting with each of the two Chiefs in the area. Discuss the program with them, and hope they will agree it would be a good thing to prevent *biri-piri* and whooping cough.

Arrange meetings throughout the District to meet with as many of the men as possible. Without their approval, we would not have success.

Pray that we find some way to obtain free measles vaccine—we couldn't afford to buy it.

Convince the hospital staff that we *had* to do this, even though they already were overworked caring for ill patients.

Train our staff on how to run a successful immunization clinic.

Pray for patience and perseverance.

Pray.

*

The answer to our prayers arrived when Dr. David Morley visited us for two days in late 1972. He was highly regarded throughout the world for programs he developed to prevent under-five mortality in developing countries. After giving him a tour of the hospital and showing him our statistics on measles, we sat on our verandah having a "sundowner." I poured my heart out to him about the preventable childhood deaths, and my frustrations and feelings of helplessness. "What can I do to vaccinate kids in this district against measles and whooping cough?"

He said, "I have a contact in London who might help. They have some nearly outdated vaccine and are interested in sending it to a rural hospital in Africa. We know that using 1/3rd dose is effective. With 2000 doses, you could vaccinate 6000 children. If you do a mass campaign, you could give vaccinations for whooping cough at the same time."

"How do I arrange for the vaccine?"

"I'll see to it. You and your staff have enthusiasm and dedication, so I'll make sure it happens." With that simple conversation, we were on the road to a vaccination program. Indeed, the Lord works in mysterious ways. Dr. Morley's insight into what it takes to be successful in less than ideal settings gave us the impetus to overcome the most difficult obstacles. He also helped obtain funding from OXFAM—Oxford Famine Relief—to help finance our "mass measles immunization campaign." God's plan was starting to work.

The next morning, Dr. Morley made rounds with me on the children's ward, and I picked his brain on how to treat various childhood diseases. Afterwards, we had tea with the staff—five German Dominican nuns, two African nuns, and two African Medical Assistant Nurses. He gave a talk about preventive medicine in the Third World, projects he had been involved with, and the good results he had seen. I knew that *if* I was to get our staff to agree to an ambitious project that was going to take several of us away from the hospital at least one day a week, someone from outside was going to have to start the process. *A prophet has no honor in his own town—Mark 6:4.* It worked. By the end of Dr. Morley's talk, there were many questions and I could see enthusiasm developing for a measles and whooping cough immunization campaign. It was no longer *my idea*, but was everyone's.

Convincing the Chiefs was easy—they knew the consequences of measles and whooping cough. Not so easy the men. I arranged to meet groups of men all over the District, taking one of the African nuns with me to speak in their native Shona language. Translated into English, a typical meeting would go like this:

"Good morning everyone. . ."

After the proper greetings, Sister would explain the vaccination program. They had *some* idea what it was about because the government held periodic polio vaccination clinics that all children were supposed to attend. Sister would ask, "Are there any questions?"

Frequently, one of the men would say, "I don't want my child vaccinated because I heard that it will make her sterile."

In some detail, Sister would reply, "The same vaccination has been used all over the world, and no one has reported any cases of infertility. It has been used in many countries in Africa, with marked decrease in measles cases." Most of the men would nod their heads in agreement, but there would still be back and forth discussions about it causing sterility. This worry about immunizations sterilizing children is still prevalent in some parts of the world today, and is hindering the worldwide project to totally eliminate polio.

A different man might then say, "I don't want my children to have measles vaccine, because if it prevents them from getting measles, they can't die from measles, and I won't know whether my wife has been unfaithful to me." A common belief held by many men was that whenever a child died—of *any cause*—it was absolute proof of his wife's infidelity. (Of course, it was mostly the men who were unfaithful and not the women.) Though many of the men believed this, they still really didn't want their children to die of measles, so other men would shout the first man down, telling him that he was a fool. Each session would take an hour or more, but by the end of the meeting, we usually had agreement that they would support our efforts and make sure their wives brought their children for the vaccinations.

One humorous episode: I was to meet a group of men who lived more than an hours drive on rough, sandy roads. Knowing that "Africa Time" was no where's near the actual time—being as much as one to two hours later—I asked the Chief to tell the men I wanted to meet them at 10:00 AM on Wednesday (I planned on being there at 11:00). The Chief, knowing his men were frequently late, told his Sub-chief to tell them they should be there at 9:00 AM. The Sub-chief, knowing his men were usually late, told them 8:00 AM. On the day of the meeting, I had an emergency Caesarean operation just as I was hoping to leave, so didn't leave until 11:00 and arrived at 12:00. Most of the men had been waiting since 8:30 or 9:00, and by then had decided I wasn't coming and went back home. *The best laid plans of mice and men* . . .

After thirty meetings with the men, we were ready to officially start the "measles campaign." The vaccine safely arrived from England, packed in dry ice. We started giving one-third dose to every new pediatric admission, abruptly stopping the "hospital contact measles." Such a relief. No longer were sick children getting measles on top of their other illness. One step completed.

Next we trained the staff and student nurses on how to weigh the children, how to give the shots, how to fill out the baby clinic cards, and how to educate mothers who had malnourished children. We first practiced with several small clinics at the hospital.

*

By June 1973, we were ready for our first clinic away from the hospital—it was up the mountain, but an easy 20-minute drive. It looked like we were going on Safari. The VW Combi (seating 12) was packed with coolers of vaccine, boxes of medicines, a balance scale for weighing babies, baby clinic cards, food for our lunch, and eight people. We drove up the rough mountain road, past our small dam, and over deep ruts in the sandy road. Just before our turnoff, we passed a woman with a baby tied on her back with a towel, and an empty fifty-gallon drum balanced on her head. I turned to Sister Perpetua and said, "Did I really see that?"

"Oh yes. That's easy, as long as the drum is empty."

Just then I turned left onto what looked like a footpath. Many thorn bushes were growing near the road. "Hope we don't get a flat tire on this road," I said.

"Oh, this road is fine," Sister replied. To her, any road you could walk on must be good enough to drive on—but then she never drove a car so she really didn't know.

"How far is it to the school?" I asked.

"It's very near." On other occasions, when I was walking somewhere and asked "How far is it to . . ." a young man would tell me, "Oh, it's very near," even when it was two or three miles. Anything less than ten miles apparently was "very near."

This time, after only two miles, we rounded a curve and came into view of the primary school where we were holding the clinic. A throng of women and children and a few men greeted us with smiles on their faces—they knew we were bringing something to prevent the scourge of measles. As we approached, the women started singing and drumming and dancing. Some of the old ambuyas (grandmothers) were ululating—the high-pitched *yeeyeeyeeyeeyee* I usually only heard in church. Such joy and happiness. I wondered, *might there have been this same atmosphere if someone had a prevention for The Black Death (Plague) during the Middle-Ages?* The sky was a deep blue with a few fluffy white clouds, but no threat of rain—a relief to us, since it meant we could hold the clinic outside under a spreading acacia tree. If it rained, we had to move inside a classroom. With kids crying and the rain drumming on the asbestos roof, the noise would be deafening. Fortunately, only a few times did we experience such a burden.

After unpacking, we set up an assembly line for weighing the children, filling out forms, a desk for me to sit where I could see each child, and finally the immunization table. Sister Perpetua gathered everyone, having them sit in a large circle. Standing just five feet tall, slightly plump, always smiling, this African nun talked to them in their native language, hands waving here and there, voice fluctuating like a practiced politician giving a political speech as she explained about the shots. She joked with them, cajoled them, shouted at them, and joked again. She involved the audience by having them repeat instructions, asking questions, and answering them. The African men and women love to talk, so sometimes she had to stop them or we would have been there all day. Finally, she gave a short talk on the prevention of malnutrition.

Then the fun began.

The long line of women, each with one or two or three children to be vaccinated, snaked into the distance and around the corner of a school building. Suckling babies, children crying, some toddlers holding onto their mothers' skirt while peering around legs to peek at us, the older ones acting nonchalant but obviously nervous about getting stuck with a needle. Because we were outside, the hubbub of noise rose into the atmosphere and was pleasurable rather than annoying—more like the pleasing babble of a rushing brook rather than the cacophony of screeching crows—which is what it sounded like when we had to hold a clinic inside.

The first woman approached the bench where we had an old-fashioned metal balance scale—a large metal pan on one side, and weights on the other. She removed the clothes from her two-year-old boy. Sister placed him on the metal pan on one side, while placing free weights on the other side, all the time helping to keep the child sitting upright in the pan. One ten-pound weight, one five-pound, a one-pound, and it balanced. "Sixteen pounds," she told the student nurse, who wrote the results on the baby-clinic card. As she removed the boy to get the next one, she noticed he had peed in the pan—a common occurrence when a bare bottom hit the cold metal. No problem. Pour it out, use the mothers' towel to wipe it dry, and ready for the next child.

The mother moved forward to sit at my table. As I perused the baby-clinic card, I could see he was four pounds below the 5th percentile for age. "What do you feed him?" I asked via my interpreter.

"*Sadza*," she replied.

"Anything else?"

"*Sadza chete*." (Only sadza, which has very little nutritional value.)

"Do you have vegetables at home?"

"Yes."

"Do you have chickens?"

"Yes."

"Do you have peanuts for making peanut butter?"

"Yes."

Turning to the student nurse interpreter, I pointed and said, "Have her go over there," where student nurses were putting on a short "drama." When they had 8 or 10 women, they would put on a 10-minute play. One would play an old Ambuya (grandmother) and the other two would play mothers with small babies:

(Shona language; much animation with finger pointing and arm waving by the actors):

First mother: *I was just listening to Sr. Perpetua, and she told me that when he turns six months, I should add one raw egg to the morning porridge. Add vegetables to the sadza afternoon and evening. Give him milk if I have it at least once a day.*

Second mother: *Yes, she also told me to use the peanuts I have to make peanut butter and add that to the porridge and sadza. If I have beans, put them in too.*

Ambuya: *No, no, no. That child only needs sadza. Listen to me. I know best.*

First mother: *But Ambuya, five of your seven children died. Maybe that wasn't the best thing to feed them?*

Ambuya: *Oh, they died from evil spirits and not because of what I fed them.*

Second mother: *Well, I have seen children that have been fed the way Sr. Perpetua says, and they all look very strong and healthy.*

Ambuya: *OK, do it your way. It's no longer like the old days where an Ambuya had some authority. Everyone has new ideas these days. Maybe it's better. I don't know.*

First and Second mothers: *Thanks, Ambuya. You're right. These are new ideas, but we need to listen to them because we want strong and healthy and smart babies.*

The observing mothers then asked questions while the student nurses continued to explain how to properly feed their children. The morality plays were well received and had a good impact on the mothers.

Nearly all families had the items mentioned, and *if* they followed the simple instructions, the child would grow at a normal growth rate. A few families were too poor to have even those items, and for those families we gave small amounts of high-protein high-calorie supplements, but most cases of malnutrition were merely ignorance of how to properly feed the child. The dramas were well received and a useful tool in educating mothers, without seeming to be lecturing them. The student nurses *loved* doing them.

Each mother then advanced to the immunization table, where the child received measles and polio and DPT vaccines—DPT is the shot for tetanus, diphtheria, and whooping cough. "One-stop-shopping for immunizations" was our goal, so each child received as many shots as possible at each clinic. We returned to the same clinic every two months, hoping that *all* children in the District would be fully vaccinated, plus it enabled us to follow children who were below weight and suggest remedies.

Slowly the undulating line advanced towards the weighing pan. Four hours later, the last child was immunized. We vaccinated 153 children for measles, and more than that for polio and DPT—we gave measles vaccine only if the child was over six months, and only if he or she had not already had measles. We finished with a feeling of accomplishment. Even though it was a lot of work, there was a carnival atmosphere. As I looked around there were smiles on everyone's face. After loading the supplies, we drove a short distance to a small flowing stream. The nursing students gathered wood for a fire and we roasted cheese sandwiches on forked sticks, ate apples, and drank lemonade for lunch—an unsurpassed banquet. I heard the student nurses talking excitedly in Shona about their experiences. Even though I couldn't understand what they were saying, it was evident it had been a great adventure.

*

One clinic completed—only 39 more to go. We developed a schedule so we would cover the entire District in a manner where no woman had to walk more than three, or at the very most, four miles. We developed an extensive communication scheme: Priests gave dates of clinics to the people at Sunday Masses, the Chief and Sub-chiefs sent messages, the teachers at each school sent the children home with the date and time several days before the event. We employed one man to work as a clerk and communicator. He rode a bicycle throughout the area a week before the clinic to inform the people. At a few clinics we had only 50 children, but at others we had 350. The average was 200. "Communication" was the key. Poor attendance wasn't because the people didn't want it, or that "they were too backward," or that their religion forbad immunizations—it was always because we hadn't communicated the event well enough. As we learned how to develop better methods of spreading the word, attendances improved.

After a nine-month campaign, the final results were rewarding: 40 clinics, over 8000 children attended, with 4100 receiving measles vaccine—the others either already had measles or were too young to vaccinate. All 8000 received DPT and polio vaccine. No serious complications were reported from the vaccinations. The following year, the hospital had 35 cases of measles, and just five deaths—compared to 150 admissions and 40 deaths the previous year. Whooping cough admissions went from 50 the previous year to 5.[2] The campaign was exhausting and became quite repetitious, with the same process over and over. Boring even. When we had the process down

---

2   I subsequently had two articles published in 1975 in the medical journal "Tropical Doctor" (United Kingdom): "*Should I do a Mass Measles Campaign*" and "*Results from a Mass Measles Immunization Campaign, Bikita District, Rhodesia.*"

pat, we combined two clinics in one exhausting day. When we analyzed the data, we all were enthused, excited, and willing to continue with Under-Five clinics as an on-going project. We realized we had much more effect on the health of the people by getting away from the hospital rather than staying at home and treating ill patients, especially true in the case of children.

Now I must develop a program to have "health scouts" live in the communities, keep records of each child's growth and development, refer cases of severe illness before the witchdoctor interferes, and try to instill good-agriculture techniques. There are government resources that might be helpful, if only we can get them to work with us rather than be suspicious of our activities. The clinics take up a lot of my time and I'm exhausted at the end of the day, especially when I have hospital emergencies to handle when we return. Still, I'm energized by the cooperation from our staff and I love getting out into the various communities to see the love and care the people have for their children and for each other. I wonder if Dr. Beth Granger, the Provincial Medical Officer, will see the benefit of our program and start supplying us with free measles vaccine?

Letter from Loretta: *October 24, 1972*

Dear Mom and Dad,

Just received your letter, and in the same mail pictures, so thought I'd get busy and send you some. We usually take slides, but were taking pictures to send with our Christmas letters. I'm still trying to persuade Dick's folks to send the negatives of our vacation to you. Apparently at some time she sent you color prints, and you didn't write to thank her, and she is a bit peeved about it.

Your Thanksgiving plans sound nice. Wish we could be there. We will have turkey and trimmings, except for pumpkin pie and cranberry sauce. None to be had here. We have invited a few Lay Mission Helpers from other missions for the weekend.

Don't worry about the package. There is a good chance they will get here by Christmas, but if they don't, I'm sure there will be something under the tree.

We finally got busy and planted some grass in our front yard, and a flowerbed. The grass is just coming up, and should be nice by Christmas. It was really a lot of work, and we did most of it ourselves. I'm beginning to enjoy gardening.

Our new puppy arrived on the 8th of this month. Her name is Suzie, is 8 weeks old, a blue eyed Dalmation. She's cute, but havoc on my two flowerbeds. She and Peter seem to be at the same stage of development. They play together, but need to be watched all the time. Suzie grabs Peter's hands, or the seat of his pants, and Peter gives her a kick now and then, but most of the time they chase each other, or a ball, and have a good time.

The weather has been hot and humid the last week. Peter and Paul had a temp. for two days, and Peter is trying to get 8 teeth all at once, so it's been miserable. Mike, Tom, and Doug had a long weekend, so I took them back to school yesterday, and brought Mary and Paul along. On the way to school, everyone began complaining about feet hurting, so I checked them at school. Mike has an ingrown toenail, badly infected, and all three have outgrown their shoes. Mary is green with envy because she heard me say we would get new ones on Friday, and she doesn't need them. She and Paul were good on the shopping trip, so we went to a tea-room for ice cream. Mary looked around and said "You know Mom, everyone in this town must be sad." I asked her why she thought that, and she said, "Look at their faces." She was right, a more sour looking group would be hard to find. Paul isn't much of a conversationalist, but he's improving, and if Mary gives him a chance to get a word in, he'll be doing OK soon.

We have a medical student from Salisbury here for two weeks. He eats with us, but sleeps at the Father 's house. He's very nice, and good company for both of us. He's getting married in December. Being around all these children has been quite an experience for him.

I began talking about the weather, yesterday guti came in, and it's really cold and drizzly. It's marvelous for the yard though. I can almost see the grass growing.

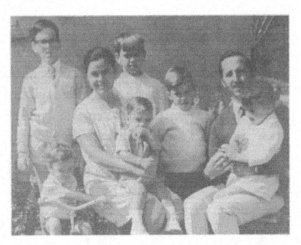

Christmas picture 1972: Mike, Paul, Loretta, Tom, Pete, Doug, Dick & Mary

Did I tell you that we've decided to send Mike to the Marist Brothers School in Que Que? It's small, about 120 students, covers 6 grades, our equivalent of high school and 2 years of Jr. College. It's multi-racial, 30% white, 20% black, and 50% Asian or mixed race (called coloreds). It means 8 hours driving on the day I pick him up or take him back. They have a month off every 3 months of school, and a 4-day weekend in the middle of each term.

We're getting our Christmas letters out now so that we can send them surface mail. I'm sending one to you so you can see how enthusiastic Dick is about his work, and something of what he is doing. We had hoped to enclose pictures, but I'm afraid they won't be ready by the last mailing date.

We are hoping to go to Gwelo on the 3rd of November to visit the Davies family. They have 6 children too. I also hope to do a little shopping. Dick is taking a Pediatric refresher course in Salisbury on Dec. 2-3, so I will get my Christmas shopping done. I need new dishes, but want a lawn mower for myself. I'm afraid that your present will be late again, as I want to get a woodcarving, and we won't be at Driefontein to buy one until some time in November.

We heard from Dick's folks that John Hart's mother passed away two weeks ago. John is married to Dick's sister Donna. His mother had an operation for a brain tumor, and just slowly went downhill from there. It has been a bad year for both of our families.

Well, best get back to my Christmas letters. Bye for now, and God bless you.

Love,

Loretta

GOD IS WITH US

February 1973:

We thought—nay, hoped?—that Peter would be our last. Good thing we didn't name him like some of the Africans do as "No More" because Loretta became pregnant again in July 1972. Since I didn't go through all those emotional rollercoaster hormonal rides, it didn't bother me, but she was unhappy at first. Then, as always, she began to enjoy the idea of another baby, *especially if it was a girl.* She and Mary began making plans and a list of names, collecting a few girl baby clothes and all the things people do to prepare for a new baby. Mary babbled away, "I just *know* this ones a girl, don't you mommy?" "Can I choose her name?" "I need to have a sister."

Towards the end of the pregnancy, it became more and more difficult for Loretta to walk down the thirty steps from our house to the lower level and up the hill to the hospital, but she and Mary needed a break from home-school classes, so every morning she brought Mary, Paul, and Peter to the hospital for morning tea. I was glad to see them each day and the three kids added spice and excitement to the talk at teatime. Mary always had a comment or two that would make the Sisters howl, and she enjoyed the attention. Peter needed constant attention or he would be under the sink, in the garbage pail, or out the door.

Paul was rambunctious and couldn't sit still during tea. One day after a few minutes he said, "Daddy, can't I go out and ride my trike?"

I was nearly finished, so said, "Yes, but stay nearby."

As I walked out of the staff room, I saw him barreling down the hill on his tricycle, totally out of control. My heart was in my throat because I could see he was going to crash into a large pile of stones. There wasn't time for me to get to him. I could only stand and helplessly watch and witness the inevitable crash, when at the last minute a student nurse whisked him off the trike, saving him from certain injury. He laughed and said, "Hi daddy. Did you see that? That was fun."

After thanking the nurse, I hugged him close to me and then scolded by saying, "Maybe you thought it was fun, but you scared me half to death. You almost ran into that pile of rocks, and then you would have been hurt bad. Don't, don't, don't ever ride your trike down that hill again. Understand?"

Meekly, "Yes, daddy."

Silveira was such a small mission that everyone would know as soon as the baby was born, so there weren't those usual questions of "Has she had the baby yet?" As soon as it came, all on the mission would know within minutes. The "bush telegraph" was efficient in such a small community.

Shortly after midnight on Wednesday February 28th, Loretta jabbed me. "Dick, get up. We have to go to the hospital."

I quickly dressed, waited for her to get ready and walked her to the hospital. On the way to the hospital I stopped at the Dominican Convent to tell Sister Rita that Loretta was in labor. After she was on the delivery bed, Sister checked her and said, "It'll be just a while. Why don't you go to your office and I'll call you when she's ready."

Thank God, the small generator was running, so we had lights. I went to my office and tried to catch up on paper work, but wasn't very successful. *Hope this goes as well as it did for Peter. Please dear God, let this be a girl. Otherwise Loretta and Mary are going to be so disappointed. I really think this will be the last—I hope—so let it be a girl. Whatever, I pray it will be healthy. Hail Mary full of grace . . .*

Two hours later Sister Rita called me, and one more time I sat at the foot of the delivery table to deliver one of our own. "Okay, the head's right here. Give me a good hard steady push."

"I am pushing. Don't tell me what to do."

"Just a bit more. There, the head has delivered. Don't push. Let me suck out the mouth."

"I have to push," and she delivered the baby with one more push. "What is it?"

"It's healthy and screaming already and has ten fingers and ten toes and is pink and has good lungs and everything's normal—but it's a boy." Such a look of disappointment.

"You promised me this one would be a girl."

"I know." What could I say? I was disappointed too, but not like she was. Boys were fine with me and we had one girl that already kept us plenty busy. Loretta was so sure this one would be a girl. She delivered seven boys and only one girl, *not fair!* But, he was healthy, which was really what we prayed for, and he would come to be loved and enjoyed and spoiled and looked after just like all the others, but for now she could be sad for a few days and wish that he was a girl.

Since there was only a large open ward on O.B. at Silveira, the Sisters made arrangements for Loretta to stay in a room at their convent. After resting a couple of hours, Sister Rita and I helped her walk the 200 yards down the hill to the convent, and for the next several days, "Sister Loretta" lived at the Dominican Convent with her bundle of joy. But, "Mom Loretta" wasn't a bundle of joy. She had real "post-partum sadness" for four days, crying a lot but still taking care of "him." Then she snapped out of it and became her normal happy motherly self.

We named him Timothy John Tinashe (God is with us) Stoughton. The Sisters teased us about "the shame descending on their convent because of baby cries emanating from within their walls and diapers hanging on the clothes line."

Loretta teased them back, saying, "You know, as a young girl I wanted to be a nun, so this is my chance. You probably won't accept me with seven children, but that might be the only way for us to not have more!"

Mary seemed to accept Timothy quicker than she did Peter. Once again she became the Big Sister who knew everything about taking care of babies, bossing the boys around on how to do this and not do that. After a week, "Sister Loretta" came home and became "just mom."

Post-script: Tim *was* the last one, and being the last, of course he was spoiled. In later years, Mary once said, "You know, Tim isn't the angel you think he is." In January 2002 we returned from our first three months back in Zimbabwe to attend his wedding to Sara, and when we returned "for good" in 2009, we stayed with them and their three children in a rental house near Tampa, Florida.

We thought it was temporary, but after we returned from visiting some of the other children, Tim and Sara said, "Come into the living room so we can have a serious talk." I thought, *Uh oh, they're sick of us being in their home and are going to ask us to look for our own place.* But no, Tim told us, "Sara and I enjoy having you living with us. It's good for our children to have their grandparents so close, and it helps us a lot. We think we should look for a house to buy, one where you could build an In-Law attachment." And that's what we did and we can recommend it to others. It's a good arrangement—the grandchildren keep us young and involved and yet we have our own space and they have their space. It's a "win-win" for all of us.

Letter from Loretta: *April 19, 1973*

Dear Mom and Dad,

I hope by now Timmy's "official" announcement has caught up to you. I'm afraid it has lost its suspense as you already know the sex.

How is Dad? Why don't you sit down and write to us Dad? How did you like trailer life and living in Mesa? Did you do much bike riding? Dick's Dad got a bicycle for his birthday. He was riding it down the street and a woman in the cafe said to the waitress who is a good friend of the Stoughton's, "Am I seeing things or did an old, gray-haired man go riding by on a bicycle?" Dick's Dad says he is going to dye his hair or get a beret.

Timmy weighted 11 lbs 4 oz on his 7-week check-up. He looks like a chipmunk. He's awake more during the day, smiles a lot, and has stopped crying in the evening.

Dick is leaving on Easter Sunday for a fishing trip with the Bishop. They are going to a very remote area on the Lundi River in one of the Game Reserves. He has been busy with so many irons in the fire since the first of the year. I'm glad he's getting away, but wish I could go too. The Bishop says this area is great: "no phone, no telegraph, no mail, . . .and no female!" The "no female" is because he spends a good bit of his time going from mission to mission in the Diocese sorting out problems with the nuns.

We're all fine except for the flu going around. The boys are enjoying no school. Peter is really a dickens. It's almost a full time job keeping up with him. The older boys went with Dick to the clinics in the airplane. Guess they didn't behave too well. Dick gave them a good talking to when they got home.

This was our announcement:

A Child Is Born:

28 February 1973; 4:21 A.M. Wt.: 8lb, 8oz

Five boys and a girl were hoping that day,
For a new baby girl, with whom all could play,
Five boys is enough for a basket ball team.
But that lonely girl! There's only a dream.

She hoped and prayed for a girl this time,
That would add some balance to this boy-girl rhyme.
A girl would be a playmate for Mary,
And some day would cause a boy to tarry.

A girl all sweet and pink and nice,
Afraid of pollywogs, snakes, and mice.
A girl to cuddle and hold so tight,
That Mary would love with all her might.

The name was ready, "Theresa Anne".
A newborn girl fulfills our plan.
Ah! Such a tale is not to be.
That newborn babe will stand to pee.
We all gather round the crib to see,
A nice healthy boy, Timothy.

Inspired by: Timothy John Tinashe (God Is With Us) Stoughton

Time to get ready for Good Friday Service. Bye for now and God Bless
you.

Love from all,

Loretta

BEWITCHED

Laurie Watts and I were on our way up the mountain to seek advice from a renowned n'anga (witchdoctor or traditional healer). He was kept busy with cases I wasn't able to cure, or more likely, with *all* the cases I treated. Most people who came to the hospital had already been to the n'anga. I certainly saw the results of those visits: multiple cut marks over the area of pain in nearly all patients; severe vomiting due to a muti (medicine) for stomach pain; occasionally complete kidney failure due to the muti; arriving very late in an illness because of the many trips to the n'anga before finally giving me a chance.

*

One day I had a conversation with one of the senior nursing students. She was quite willing to talk openly about practices of the traditional healer and the beliefs of her rural people, *as long as we were alone.* I asked her, "Why do so many people visit the n'anga before coming to see me?"

"It's complicated. But mostly it's so that any difficulties with the ancestors are resolved."

"Difficulties with the ancestors?"

She looked around to see if anyone was listening. "Imagine that I have done something that would upset my dead grandfathers' spirit. It would then have an influence on my health and I might develop headaches."

"What would upset him?"

"Oh, just about anything. Talking with a boy he might not like. Not walking home on a weekend to see my father. Not studying hard enough."

"And how would the n'anga put things right?"

Looking off into the distance, she paused and said, "First I have to pay him. Then he'll go through a process to communicate with my grandfather's spirit, and finally he'll try to convince my grandfather that I'm sorry and will do better. Then he'll tell me what I have to do in the future."

Since she wore a small cross on a chain, I asked her, "Are you Catholic?"

"Oh, yes."

"Sounds a bit like confessing to a priest."

"It is a bit, but it's also different. For example, he might give me some medicine to help with the pain, or he might give me some advice on how to keep my grandfather happier. But what he does best is to make things right with my grandfather's spirit."

"After leaving him, do you feel better and does the headache go away?"

"Yes."

"Have you been to one?"

"Many times."

"You're a smart young woman. You've studied nursing so you know about the causes of pneumonia?"

"Of course."

"If you had pneumonia and knew that penicillin would cure it, would you still go to the n'anga?"

Again she looked nervously around to see if anyone else was there. "Sure."

"If you knew that penicillin would cure it, why see the n'anga?"

She looked at me as if I was really stupid and didn't understand what she had just explained. She said, "Oh, but the question is *why* did I get pneumonia? Maybe it was because my grandfather was upset. I have to resolve that issue with him or the penicillin might not work, or else I'll soon get another illness that might be worse."

"Are you nervous talking to me about this?"

Shyly, "Just a bit. It sort of feels like I'm giving away some secrets, even though I know I'm not. Some of my classmates might not like it."

I learned that the ancestors always have to be placated. To me it seemed like good psychological counseling and maybe that was "the good" the n'anga could do. If only they would stick to the psychological side of it. My problem was that he or she many times gave exactly the wrong medicine and made the person with real medical problems worse instead of better. I hoped that our visit to a real live n'anga would shed some light on his practices.

I had a case where he had dramatic results. Eighteen-year-old Faith had delivered her first baby, a healthy 7-pound boy. Problems developed on the second day when she was unable to breast-feed. In the U.S. we would tell the mother, "Well, for this first baby it looks like you'll need to feed formula," and that would solve the problem. It was a huge problem for Faith, because without breast milk her baby boy would die, since she couldn't afford formula. In addition, there was the common belief that being unable to breastfeed was absolute proof she had been unfaithful to her husband. This "unfaithfulness" could entail something as innocent as Faith looking at a good-looking guy and thinking about him. It didn't require any physical action; not even a coy smile. It was hard for me to believe, but there it was and there was nothing I could do. We tried everything to help Faith, all to no avail. Finally, on the fourth day she was missing from the ward, her baby still asleep in the bassinette.

I asked the ward nurse, "Where's Faith?"

"We think she went to visit the n'anga."

Later that day she returned with a smile on her face, picked the baby up and started to nurse him. Success! Of course, I believed the n'anga had relieved her anxiety in some manner and that allowed her milk to come. The baby could sense his mother was no longer nervous and anxious and quickly latched onto a breast and started sucking. I didn't try explaining my theory to the student nurses—they wouldn't have believed me.

We frequently had patients who thought they had been bewitched, but recently there had been a flurry of activity, with three other cases. One was a very young woman who was sure the spirit of her father was making her ill. She had been to several n'angas with no relief. Unless her belief could be cured, I was sure her headaches would continue, and I'm afraid we didn't have much success. Another was a young boy who had been seen many times for abdominal pain. The n'anga told him that the father's sister bewitched him. For that reason, his entire family moved away from where the aunt lived! The aunt might not even know anything about it.

Innocent was a man dying from malignant melanoma. The family discussed it with the Chief, and the Chief somehow decided a certain neighbor man was bewitching Innocent. The accused man even admitted to it—maybe he had some "bad thoughts" about Innocent—and now he had to work to pay for the hospital fees. Explaining to them that this was a cancer and not caused by any "spirits" didn't help, because they answered, "Yes, but why did he get that cancer in the first place? That is where the spirit was involved." How could I argue against that?

*

Laurie, who had been with us for two weeks, was leaving in a couple of days, and it was at his request that we were driving up the mountain. He had seen all of the above cases, and wanted to see a witchdoctor before he left. He was a fourth-year medical student from McMasters University in Canada, but his home was in Trinidad, and he was black. It was only by the mismanagement of a Rhodesian white bureaucrat that Laurie was in the country. He was accepted for a two-month clerkship at Harare Hospital in Salisbury without anyone in immigration seeing a picture of him. They just assumed that being from a Canadian medical school, he must be white. Laurie told me the story about arriving at the airport: An immigration agent looked at him and said, "But you're black."

With a deadpan expression, Laurie said, "Yes, I know."

"But, but—you're not supposed to be allowed in the country. We don't allow blacks from other countries."

"I didn't know that. I have a valid visa."

"I see that. What am I to do?"

"Let me in. I won't cause any problems. Promise."

"I don't know." He furtively looked around hoping to find someone to help him. When no one came, he finally said, "Oh Hell, here you are," stamped the passport and waved him through. After six weeks at Harare Hospital, Laurie arranged to spend his last two weeks with us. Before leaving Silveira, he wanted to visit a n'anga, and since I had been wanting to as well, I arranged it through the Headman (local leader) who lived at the top of the mountain.

*

Two miles up the mountain road I stopped at Benny's homestead. He was one of my "health scouts"—men we had trained to ride bicycles throughout the district in the manner of the "barefoot doctors" in China. It was another of our attempts to get the hospital out into the community. The health scouts were having great success and Benny was at the head of the class.

After the usual greeting, I said to Benny, "We want to visit the Headman up at the top of Denga. He told me there was a famous n'anga there that we want to see."

Benny had a quizzical look on his face. "Why do you want to go all the way up there? I have several nhangas here."

"No, the Headman said I should go to his place and he would take me there. Come with us to show the way."

Benny climbed into the backseat and we wound our way up the mountain to near the top. Henry, the Headman for that area, came to greet us. We sat on stumps of wood and Benny, speaking in Shona, proceeded to tell Henry that we wanted to see his pumpkins. Henry, knowing we were there to visit the n'anga, shook his head and said, "No, they want to see the n'anga, not some nhangas." The two of them rolled back and forth laughing so hard they nearly fell on the ground. I thought I might have to treat them for a stroke.

Of course, all of this conversation was in Shona, so Laurie and I wondered what was so hilarious. They finally stopped laughing and Benny was able to control himself long enough to explain that "n'anga" is pronounced with an implosive swallowing sound after the "n." I had been pronouncing it as *nhanga* (naanga or "a" like baa), and *nhanga* means pumpkin. Benny thought I wanted to see a famous pumpkin. Again they were off in gales of laughter, and Laurie and I couldn't help but join in making fun of the doctor and his (lack-of) Shona. After all, if you can't laugh at yourself, you shouldn't laugh at others. What a story they could tell everyone about the Chiremba (doctor) and his sad attempts at speaking Shona, turning a witchdoctor into a pumpkin.

We finally stopped laughing enough for Henry to lead us down a narrow path. Goats and chickens scattered in front of us, a couple of cows were munching on the sparse grass, two goats were chasing the chickens, and we arrived at a very average looking rural African compound. It overlooked a drop-off towards the South, with scattered villages seen far in the distant haze. A cool breeze wafted over us, carrying smoke from a wood fire up the mountain. There were four round huts with grass-thatched roofs. Sitting by the fire was a bare-chested, middle-aged man wearing ragged brown shorts. He rose to greet us, and Henry introduced us to Magazine Bhebhe, the famous n'anga, who didn't look at all like a pumpkin but also didn't look like a famous witchdoctor. Henry explained to Mr. Bhebhe that we were there for a "professional visit," and wanted a consultation. The charge was one shilling—about 15 cents. After paying him, he excused himself to go into his hut where he put on his regalia.

Emerging from the hut, he was transformed into what I imagined a n'anga might look like: Dressed in several leopard skins, a headdress of feathers and bright ribbons, and carrying a variety of whistles, bones, dice, and a mirror. He spread two large zebra skins on the ground for us to sit on, and I had Benny interpret for us. We didn't tell Mr. Bhebhe what ailment we had or why we were there—he just started.

He began with chanting and shaking a gourd filled with pebbles, his shoulders moving up and down in tune to the chant. His voice modulated high and then low, he grabbed a whistle and blew several short blasts, then a different high-pitched whistle (I later learned this was to get the attention of the spirits). More chanting, more whistling, louder and louder to a frenzy, and suddenly stopped. He threw a few small bones onto the skins, looked in the mirror, threw the dice, looked in the mirror, blew the whistle, and said, "You are having headaches."

We answered, "No." That didn't bother him at all. Laurie and I wondered why not? We would be upset if we told a patient they had one thing and they answered "No I don't." We asked Benny, and he explained that the n'anga was visualizing a "continuum" of time—past, present, and future. It didn't matter to him that what he saw was not in the present—he would eventually find the right time frame.

With a nearly blank expression on his face, he began the same process, with even louder chanting and whistling, more shaking his shoulders up and down, seemingly even more in a trance. He again threw the bones and then the dice and looked into the mirror and blew the whistle and shook the rattles and chanted and suddenly stopped: "You are having stomach problems."

"No."

Same process. "You lost some money."

"No."

No change in his expression. He started all over again, repeated the chant, the whistles, the bones, the mirror: "You are going on a long journey and are worried about it."

Well, Laurie was flying back to Canada in a few days but he wasn't worried, so we replied, "No."

"You are having problems with your wife."

"No." I better not admit to that!

"You're having chest pains and cough."

'No." Since we really hadn't gone to see him for a specific problem, he didn't hit on any of our concerns, but that didn't bother him. He would have continued for more of the same if we hadn't stopped him.

We realized he had a set number of maladies to "cure," and most of the people coming to him would indeed have one of them. They might then exclaim to a neighbor, "He *knew* I was going on a journey and was worried about it. He took care of my conflict with Uncle Joe's spirit, and now I can travel without worry."

We had a few questions for him: "How did you get to be a n'anga?"

"My father was a famous n'anga for many years. When he died, the family gathered here for his funeral." He stood, pointed to a large forested area and continued, "After the funeral, we all went into that forest to see who would find his spirit. I wandered there for several hours and found it, so I became the n'anga."

"How did you know you found his spirit?"

"I just knew it and so did everyone else."

"Did you have any training?"

Shaking his head sideways he said, "Only by watching my father when I was a child." *Hmm. Not at all like our Native American Medicine Men who spend years in training with older and wiser Healers.*

"What do you give a child with diarrhea?"

He went into the hut and brought out a small gourd filled with a clear fluid. "What is this?"

He showed us some beans that looked like castor beans. So, the treatment for diarrhea was to give the person—adult or child—castor oil, something that would make it worse. Not much different than when our grandmothers gave "a good dose of the salts (Epsom salts)" to really clean you out if you had diarrhea. I thought, *I must see if I can get our Health Scouts to gingerly and cleverly try to change a few of the n'anga's practices.*

"What do you use for headache?"

Now he looked all around to be sure no one else was there. Finally he reached into a pocket and brought out something that looked very much like ground-up daga, or marijuana. Laurie and I nodded wisely and thought, *That should do the trick. Not in my arsenal though.*

We thanked Mr. Magazine Bhebhe, walked back up the slope to our car, and drove down the mountain. Maybe I heard the Headman still laughing at us while we drove off? *Imagine not knowing the difference between a pumpkin and a witchdoctor.*

SEE ST. PETER?

I was on my "flying doctor" trip of four clinics in three days, only this month it was totally upside down. First of all, I started on Monday rather than Wednesday, and then I had to do the four of them in just two days, because Brother John—who flew the plane to Silveira—was going fishing with the Bishop and was leaving early Wednesday morning. Secondly, I had two passengers: Sister Laetitia—one of our African Nuns—and Brother Bruno. Sister wanted to experience the flying trip and clinic visits, and Brother Bruno was learning to fly so he could help Brother John. We hoped this trip would be good experience for him.

Matibi Clinic was very quiet and I was finished in an hour, so we made the five-minute flight across the Lundi River to Berejena, landing at 10:00 AM. Although only a five-minute flight, the two Clinics were over 100 miles apart by road. The Lundi river was impassable for most of the year, so despite the close proximity, they were hours apart by foot or car. They were expecting us at Berejena, but that morning there wasn't a car or truck at the mission. After waiting 15 minutes, Sister Margaret arrived with a Scotch Cart—a two-wheeled cart pulled by a donkey. We came by airplane to the airstrip and then by donkey cart to the Mission—where else but in Africa could that happen? We all piled into the cart and bumped our way to the Mission.

Sister Margaret first took me to see a woman bleeding from an incomplete miscarriage. Sister didn't know what to do. I said to her, "Why don't you do a D&C?"—a procedure to scrape the inside of the uterus to get rid of the remaining tissue that was causing the bleeding.

"I've never done one. Why don't you and Sister Laetitia do it for me?"

"No, you can do it, and then if a case like this comes in again, you can do it without a problem. It's a simple operation and you only need to use a bit of IV pain medicine."

I proceeded to talk her through the D&C. She held the curette tentatively at first, but eventually learned what it felt like to be gentle and yet firm in scraping the inside of the uterus. Finally there was no more tissue to be scraped and the bleeding stopped. With a smile she turned to me and said, "That wasn't so difficult. Thanks for showing me."

"You're most welcome." It was such a pleasure for me to see someone at these clinics that was eager to learn and wanted to be able to do new procedures. *Sister, you just made my day. Maybe my worries about the out-lying clinics being resistant to change was not such a big problem after all.*

I finished seeing patients at 12:30. A car had returned to the Mission and could drive us to the plane, so we decided to fly to St. Peter's that afternoon. A few low-lying clouds might make the trip interesting. Halfway to St. Peter's it was more interesting than I wanted. The clouds drifted lower and lower, and soon I couldn't see the tops of the surrounding hills. I climbed above the clouds. *Is this a good idea? What would your flying instructor say? "Turn around, go back where you came from, and wait for the weather to clear." That's what he would say, but did I listen? No.* I wrongly thought that if I was on top of the clouds, I would see a clearing to the East and would be able to land at St. Peters. I saw one opening, went down through it only to find the surrounding hills still covered with clouds, so back up again we went. This time, in order to not be in clouds and maybe hit one of those hills, I had to make a tight climbing turn. Sister Laetitia didn't like it one bit. I thought she might be thinking we were going to see "Saint Peter at the Pearly Gates" rather than get to St. Peter's Mission on the Sabi River. Did I really hear her start saying a "Hail Mary?" Once back on top, there were solid clouds to the east as far as the eye could see. It was clear to the north, so I tuned in the navigation signal from Fort Victoria and we headed there. Just over the airport was a lovely opening—thank God—and I landed. One hour of flight time and no closer to our destination. I heaved a sigh of relief to be safely on the ground, turned to Bruno and said, "Brother Bruno, that is *not* the way to fly in bad weather."

"I thought you did a good job. What's the problem?"

"No, I should have stayed under the clouds and turned back to Berejena as soon as they started closing in. That's the thing to do, and remember that. I was really lucky to find such a big hole right over this airport."

We waited two hours, the weather cleared, the report was good all the way to St. Peter's, so once again we were on our way with two hours of daylight remaining. I flew over the Mission several times, but since they weren't expecting me until the next day, we were ignored. I landed and we waited, wondering if we were going to have to walk the three miles to the clinic, when a pickup truck from the irrigation scheme drove by. A young man called out, "Hey Doc, you need a ride?"

"Sure do. Thanks," and he drove us to the clinic. Brother Bruno went off to do some maintenance work at the mission while Sister Laetitia stayed with me to see the clinic.

Kay and Annette were still at the clinic and surprised to see us. "You weren't supposed to be here until morning."

"I know, but I'm hoping to get an early start tomorrow so I can get back to Silveira by early afternoon. This is Sister Laetitia. How are you all?"

"Hi Sister. Yah, we're busy as Hell. Malaria season is here. Last month we had over a thousand cases, with 3000 outpatient visits."

"That means 100 every day of the month. How do you do it?"

"Vell, it keeps us out of trouble."

*

Kay Von Dudekom, a lay-missionary from Los Angeles, was a large Dutch-American woman with a strong accent. She was a registered nurse and the only qualified medical person for the entire area. The nearest hospital was 160 miles away. Her lay-missionary assistant, Annette Corpron, was a petite blond physical therapist, not even a trained nurse. But, with all the nursing and medical treatments that Kay taught her over the previous three years, she worked alongside Kay just like a nurse. Lay Mission Helpers Association in Los Angeles—a Sister organization to Mission Doctors Association—trained them and sent them to Rhodesia. They worked well together and were an inspiration for me. *Why couldn't Dr. George and I get along like this? What's the matter with us?*

St. Peter's Mission was right on the banks of the Sabi River. During the night, hippos came out of the river to eat the vegetables in their garden. Occasionally, when called at night, they had to take care not to bump into a hippo as they walked up the road to the clinic. They even had names for them: Hilda the Hippo, Humphrey the Hippo, etc. Luckily, those hippos were more interested in the vegetables than they were in Kay or Annette, because hippos can be dangerous as I chronicled in the chapter, "Barking Dog."

"Do you have any in-patients I should see tonight?"

"Yah, let's make rounds on all of them. Here's a tiny one with tetanus. He's now two weeks old and slowly improving."

Gazing at the tiny, wrinkled two-week old infant, I inquired, "What are you treating him with?"

"Mostly good nursing care, but also Penicillin and some tiny doses of Valium to help with seizures. He's much better today and I think he's going to make it." Tetanus of the newborn was fairly common around St. Peter's because most deliveries were at home, and it was customary to rub dung onto the severed umbilical cord to ward off evil spirits. Of course, the dung carried the tetanus organisms and *if* the mother had not been immunized against tetanus, then the baby was apt to get it. Even with the best of care, neonatal tetanus had a high mortality rate, but Kay and Annette were able to save nearly 50% of their cases with their excellent nursing care, even to the extent of sometimes taking the baby home with them during the night. An easy prevention was to immunize all pregnant mothers against tetanus, and then the mother's antibodies protect the newborn infant. Since most delivered at home, they also didn't come for antenatal care, so no tetanus shots. Women of childbearing age who came to the clinic for any reason were given a tetanus shot, with the theory that it didn't do any harm and would do a world of good if she became pregnant.

The women's ward was filled with malaria cases, most of them improving and nearly ready for discharge, even with blood counts one-third of normal. Malaria destroys red blood cells and people with chronic malaria get used to very low blood counts. The men wouldn't allow their wives to stay in the clinic for more than two or three days, so it was fortunate that with treatment, malaria victims quickly improved, even in the most severe cases. On the male ward was a man with cerebral malaria who was agitated and thrashing about. "Do you have any more valium?" I asked.

"Yah, we have a small supply."

"Let's give him 5 mg. I.V. and see how he does."

After finishing rounds, we walked to their house for supper, a glass of wine, and plenty of talk about their work, their worries, and their plans.

"Any interesting cases, lately?" I asked.

"Just the usual, but we did have an interesting experience last week," said Kay.

"What was that?"

"Yah, the Wild Game Officers in this area determined that there were way too many hippos for the area. They were coming out of the river and destroying crops and endangering the people."

"Yes, you told me about nearly bumping into one when going to the clinic in the middle of the night."

"Yah, that was Hilda. But she's gentle and no problem. Some of the others were much more aggressive and had to be culled. We were sorry to hear they were going to do it, but understood the reasoning."

Annette went on, "Before dawn the day of the culling, we drove to the area where they were going to do it. They had already notified the local people where and when it would be done, so there were at least 200 Africans quietly mulling about nearby. The three hippos had just finished their night-time foray into the maize fields, and just as the sun came up, they were seen slowly ambling back towards the river."

Kay continued: "Suddenly there were three loud shots, and all three hippos fell where they stood. The Rangers went to each one and put a bullet into their brains to make sure they were dead, then stepped back and let the local people have at it."

Annette: "And have at it they did. It was unbelievable. There was a loud scream as the men surrged forward with sharp pangas (long knives). They lunged at the hippos, with the fastest ones slicing into the belly and diving inside to get the choice parts—liver and spleen and heart. They emerged full of blood and gore, but with wide smiles as they held up their treasures."

Kay: "Within fifteen minutes, nothing was left of any of the hippos except a blood stain on the ground. Not even any bones. All the parts were rapidly cut and distributed, with no arguing or complaining. A long line of women walked away with large pans balanced on their heads, happily singing that there would be meat on the fire that day. The men followed, strutting like hunters returning from a successful hunt."

And that was the sad but exciting ending to three marauding hippos.

"I wish I had been there. Did you get any pictures?"

"Unfortunately, no. The authorities didn't want any pictures because they feared animal activists might cause trouble."

"Changing the subject, Annette, when are you leaving?"

"In just four months. I'll be sorry to go, and especially sorry to leave Kay alone, but I'm ready to be back in the U.S. and see my family."

So far there was no replacement coming from Los Angeles for Annette. I didn't think Kay could manage being alone in such an isolated place, but she said she would stick it out for another year to see if anyone else came. Annette did return to L.A. and shortly afterwards was diagnosed with Hodgkin's Lymphoma, dying just a few years later.

The next morning I finished by seeing some outpatients with them. They really didn't need my help because they were the experts and I was the student. By noon it was time to leave and Annette drove us to the airstrip. Giving her a hug, I wished her well, invited them to drive to our place the next month to spend a long weekend, and took off into the wind. I made a turn to fly over the clinic, waggled my wings to Kay who was waving outside the clinic. As I turned towards Mukaro Clinic, I thought "*What a job those two are doing. They fill me with awe. They're the true missionaries, living in much poorer conditions than we do, bringing love and care to the poorest of the poor, and doing it with such happiness and determination. It's a privilege to be associated with them. Our Mission Rings say, "For We Are God's Helpers; Heal The Sick." They do that in spades and do it with such love and compassion. Now if I can only find Mukaro without problem and get through the patients quickly so I can get back to Silveira in time to take care of any new problems that have arrived.*

Letter from Loretta: *Oct. 14, 1973*

Dear Mom and Dad,

I just finished a letter to you, but Dick and I have just had a serious talk, and made a decision, so I have to throw that one away, and start a new one. It seems M.D.A. has no new doctors to come next summer, and Dick feels he needs one more year to really get his program well established, plus he has some new ideas for things to get started. Much of his work will be wasted if we leave in July '74 and no doctor comes to replace us, so we have written to M.D.A. and asked if they would send us home for a 2-month leave starting the beginning of this December, and in return we would stay till July of 1975, with the possibility open to stay till '76. In many ways it's a good idea for us. We would spend December in Iowa and January in S.D., with Dick traveling around to propagandize for recruits for M.D.A. and to look at places we might be interested to live when we do get back.

It means that Mary would spend 6 months in boarding school, which will be hard on her, but she's pretty wild, and the discipline would be helpful for her. I hate to put her right into an American school where there is so little discipline. Also, I would like to teach Paul. I think that giving that much of my time without having competition from the others would be good for him. For my own self, it would be hard to get along without the help of the girls while the children are so young . It will be four weeks before we hear the answer, but I wanted to let you know so you could make plans for us to be home in January. I am so excited at the thought of coming home, and hope so much that it will happen.

Timmy has gone from "easy to care for" stage to the "frustrated, wanting to do more than he can" stage. He's trying hard to stand, but our furniture has few handholds. He manages to pull himself in his bed. He goes all over in his walker, and loves his little jumper swing. He looks like a

Jack in the Box jumping up and down. Paul's getting to the philosophical stage. He's asked me "When will we see God" every day for the last week.

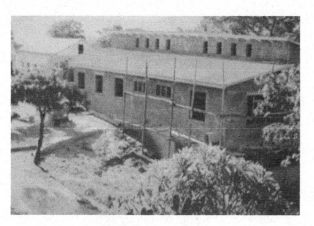

New hospital under construction

We are expecting two medical students from Salisbury on the 22nd. They'll be here for two weeks. Dick always enjoys having them. The hospital building is coming along. We have moved into a few rooms already. What will hold us up is the cabinetry—there is so many needed for the Lab., OR, Drug Room and Sterilizing room. Perhaps it will be finished by the time we get back from the U.S. Dick's Measles Campaign is going well. We have not had a case from this area, but have had a few from another reserve. Dick has arranged to do a few clinics in that area now. We have had a few cases of Malaria from very close by, so we're being very careful to take our Malaria pills.

Thank you for getting the presents in the mail. We may have them for Valentine's Day. We have all agreed that going home will be the best present we can have for Christmas. I guess it will be New Years we will be spending with you, but it will all be Christmas to us. I am so happy thinking about it.

Well, it's getting late, so I will say bye for now. God bless you all.

Love, Loretta

WORRY, WORRY, WORRY

February 1975:

10:00 PM: It was as black as the inside of a cave on a moonless night, a driving rain was lashing our roof, and I was worried. Loretta wasn't back from taking the boys to the Marist Brothers boarding school near Que Que. It was a 4-hour drive each way. She left at 7:00 that morning and should have been home hours ago. *Where is she?* There were rumors of terrorist activity near the borders, but nothing in the interior of the country. The thought of terrorism lurked in the back of my mind like a mouse gnawing on a string. The later it got, the more that mouse gnawed off the sting and the more worried I became. *This "terrorist war" is getting worse. Why can't they use Gandhi's method of non-violence? That worked. Black rule is inevitable. Twenty Blacks to one White means it will happen some day—sooner rather than later. Why can't the White's see that? Are they really that dense? The Black's want more presence in the government, but the White's always give "too little too late." If only they would develop a strategic plan towards majority rule within a reasonable period of time, then the violence would stop. Now both sides are killing innocent people who have no part in the struggle other than being of the "wrong color in the wrong place at the wrong time." Neither side has much concern for innocent lives being lost. Where will it all end? What will we do if the struggle comes to this area?*

It was raining so hard it would be difficult for Loretta to drive on our rough, sandy road. The small streams could even be in flood and she might not be able to get across the "under-water bridges"—the cement slabs in low spots of the road to prevent washout during the rainy season. From our living room window, I could see a two-mile stretch of road that approached the mission. The kids were long asleep and I was keeping a lonely vigil, nervously pacing back and forth in the living room, one candle burning on the dining table as I peered out the window into the black gloomy night, hoping to see the lights of a car, praying that she was alright. All I saw were flashes of lightning and then pure blackness. No way for me to call someone to find out, and probably no way for her to call me. Even if she tried to call, the one mission phone at the hospital was usually out of order. Just for something to do, I went down to talk with Father Kilchmann and Brother Serafin. They tried to assure me that she was probably okay, but I could see they too were worried. It was raining too hard for anyone to take a vehicle out to the main road, and anyway, what good would that do? All I could do was wait and pray.

11:00 PM: Still no evidence of a car on the road. Once more I went down and talked with Brother Serafin. We could only surmise what might have happened. Maybe she decided it was too late and stayed at the parish house in Fort Victoria? Since the phone didn't work, we wouldn't know until morning. He knew I was worried and so was he, but what could we do?

I said, "Should we try to drive out to the main road?"

Brother Serafin said, "We might not even get across the river near the mission, so let's wait another hour. If she's not here by then, we'll see if we can get across." I went back up to our house and continued praying and pacing and peering into the blackness of the night and the rain.

Midnight: Yes! Finally, there were lights of a car slowly snaking along the winding road towards the mission. Worried about the stream near the mission being in flood, I ran down the hill to the entrance of the mission. Outside the gate, the usually tiny stream was in full flood, with water rushing at least a foot or more over the bridge. Just as I arrived, the VW Van appeared on the other side. Loretta got out and waved and shouted, but with the rain and the roar of the stream, I couldn't hear a thing. I waved that she should stay there and not try to cross. We would have to wait until the water went down or the van might be carried away. She sat in the van as I waited in the rain. Brother Serafin arrived, and together we tried to gauge when it might be safe to walk across the bridge and help drive the car to the mission. The rain lessened and by 12:45 AM the water was low enough for me to gingerly ease my way onto the cement platform, and step-by-step cautiously inch my way across the bridge, water swirling to my knees. Loretta got out and with rain streaming down our faces, we hugged and kissed and hugged again.

"Oh, am I glad to see you. What a day I've had."

"I was so worried. Why are you so late?"

"It's a long story. Let's go home. I'll take a hot shower and then tell you about it."

I carefully drove the car across the steam, safely reaching the other side without incident, and we proceeded to our house. After her shower, we sat together in the living room with a cup of hot coffee with a shot of brandy, and she told me her story:

"I'm sorry for all the concern I've caused you and everyone else, dear. I know how it worries you when I'm late. Thank goodness I didn't bring any of the young ones with me. I did try to phone but couldn't get through. Let me begin at the beginning. We had an uneventful trip to Que Que. I drove the Gwelo way, as I know you prefer me to go that way, and we had time to get the boys settled before lunch. The Brothers invited me to eat with them. By the way, everyone sends you greetings. There were no errands to run in town, so I decided to make the trip shorter by taking the gravel road to Umvuma. How I wish I hadn't. After a while the car became difficult to steer, so I stopped to look at the tires. The back left one was flat. I've watched you change flats, so thought I could do it myself. I found the instruction book in the glove compartment, but it was in German. Still, the pictures were clear enough, so I took out the spare and the tools, jacked up the car and got the hubcap off, but then, no matter how hard I tried, I couldn't get the lugs loose. I was so mad that I didn't have the strength to do it. I had been so proud of myself up to that point.

Then it started raining. I was parked on one of those darned under-water bridges, so I had to take the jack off and drive the car to higher ground, and then started to walk—and walk—and walk. Unfortunately, I hadn't worn my running shoes, but had on the strappy sandals I wear for dress shoes. I knew it was at least seven miles to the main road—maybe more—but it didn't look like anyone would come on the gravel road, so off I went. It rained off and on and then the sun would come out. It was a beautiful area for a walk, but I hope I never have to do it again.

There were a few trees near the road, and I crossed to whichever side they were on in order to walk in the shade. There were many monkeys and baboons. The only time I was scared was when I came upon a herd of Brahmin cattle in the field near the road. I could see at least one bull. Having watched how fierce Brahma bulls were in rodeos, it made me uneasy to see them so near the road, and the dumb things started to follow me. I didn't want to throw a rock and get them mad, so I just walked fast and left them behind. Since it was such a long walk, I had lots of time to think, and started to think about the reports of terrorists in the country. Of course, terrorists in the country didn't mean in that area, so I talked myself out of that worry. I pulled out my Rosary, and saying the prayers helped.

My watch was at home, so I had no idea of the time, but the sun was getting lower in the sky. On the horizon were trees going in a line perpendicular to the road I was on, so I hoped they were on the main road. They were, but it was nearly dark by the time I reached it. I began walking along that road to Umvuma, still a few miles away. Fortunately, a farmer in a pickup stopped to ask why I was walking on the road at that time of night, and I explained my situation. He was shocked that I had walked so far by myself, and offered me a ride to the garage. Arriving just before closing time, the manager had one of his workers drive me back to the Combi and change the tire. Then we drove back to the shop where they insisted the flat tire be fixed before I go any farther. I tried to phone the mission from there, but couldn't get through.

After the tire was fixed, it was quite dark as I began my journey home, but I was so exhausted from my long walk that I started to fall asleep at the wheel. After nearly running off the road, I pulled over at a Rest Area to take a short nap. I leaned my head against the wheel and when I woke and looked at the dashboard clock, I saw I had slept nearly two hours. By this time it had started to rain again. Because of the rain, it was slow, even on the good road. It was raining much harder when I turned onto our road at 11:00. It was even more difficult driving, and I had to drive in second gear and sometimes in first. The first two underwater bridges had water over them, but I was able to get across. I was so glad to see you at the last one because I don't know what I would have done if you weren't there."

"What a day. I was so happy to see those lights coming towards the mission. You can imagine how worried I was. From now on we're going to have someone go with you on that trip. It's just too dangerous for you being alone and too worrisome for me."

"I won't mind having someone along. It's such a long drive to make by myself. How much longer are we going to be here?"

"I know you and the kids are ready to be back in the States, but I can't leave until there's a replacement. We've done too much work to just leave without someone to carry on the programs we started. Mission Doctors has promised to have someone within the next year."

"Yes, I know. Most of the time I'm really happy here, but when something like this happens, I keep wishing we were back home someplace, wherever that someplace might be."

With that, we finished our coffee and settled into our warm bed, happy to have each other to snuggle against. "Goodnight dear. I'm glad you're safely home."

"Me too."

Is this a warning? I was so worried that something bad had happened to her, that maybe those terrorists incidents weren't only on the borders. With the tensions increasing, maybe I have to start thinking seriously about leaving even if there isn't a replacement? I would never forgive myself if something happened to Loretta or to some of the kids. Our work here is important and fulfilling, but safety of our family comes first. What to do. What to do. Maybe Mission Doctors will have someone who will be coming in the next few months . . .

Letter from Loretta: *March 1, 1975*

Dear Mom and Dad,

I'm only a little late this time. Hope you had a happy birthday Mom, and a nice anniversary.

We had a very nice week in Malawi, where we had to go for our passport renewals. The weather was bad, so we flew Commercial rather than take the Cessna. One of the Marist Brothers met us at the airport, drove us around on our business, arranged for a place for us to stay, and took us out to dinner. He was a very entertaining host, and we had a grand time. Next day we got our passports, did some shopping, and then took a bus to Likuni Mission, a five-hour ride. We have a Mission Doctor there, and four Lay Mission Helpers, so we enjoyed our visit. We toured Lilongwe, the new capital of Malawi, and it is beautiful. We took the bus back to Zomba and stayed at the Marist Brothers house. Next day we went in to Blantyre and flew home. We enjoyed every minute. We arrived back home in Silveira about 11:00 p.m. Monday evening. Everything went on fine without us; the children were good, etc. We had a royal welcome from them the next morning.

Tim had his second birthday the 28th. The whole mission staff came up for cake and ice cream. We drank 4 bottles of wine. It was a pretty good party for a two year old. Now Peter and Paul are looking forward to their birthdays. They both want the same thing, a baby cat with a mother cat. We already have that combination, but each one wants his very own. Mary is worse—she wants a pony.

We have had bad news from M.D.A. Maybe I already told you, the doctor we expected is not coming. We are writing everywhere: England, Germany, Switzerland, and the U.S. I don't expect that we will leave by August, but I hope by December. If no one is coming, I am not sure that

Dick will leave. The boys don't seem to mind at all. I thought they would be very disappointed, glad they're not.

Could you do a favor for me and send us a Barbie doll and some clothes for it? I hope it will be an acceptable substitute for a horse for Mary. Thanks.

Love from all, Loretta

DIFFICULT TIMES REQUIRE
NEW STRATEGIES

September, 1975:

Towards the end of our time at Silveira, I was increasingly concerned with the possibility that the civil war was going to gradually come to our mission. One of my biggest concerns was what would they do for women who needed C-sections? There might not be a doctor because of the danger, and if the war caused restrictions on normal road travel, women and babies might die due to the lack of a surgeon.

At a staff meeting with only the nuns present, I said to them, "I think I should train one of you to do C-sections."

They all looked at me, shaking their heads back and forth, indicating "Not me." Then Sister Rosemary pointed to Sister Perpetua and said, "She could do it."

"Oh no, not me. I couldn't do that. Never," said Perpetua.

She had been my assistant for many operations, including countless C-sections, and I knew she had the talent and ability to do them *if* she had more training and could gain confidence. A C-section is really an easy operation if you know how to stay out of trouble. I said to her, "I think you can. You just need more training."

During normal times, the Ministry of Health would never have allowed non-doctors to do surgery, but those were not normal times. The coming war years might sever connections from all hospitals, so a different strategy was needed.

Sister Perpetua wasn't even a Registered Nurse—she was a "medical assistant," trained in our school. Barely 5 feet tall (if that), she needed a step stool when assisting me; otherwise, she could barely see over the abdomen.

The two of us went into the operating room. With the surgical book open, I walked her step-by-step through a normal C-section. She knew all the steps, but if she was going to do them, she needed to know them inside-out and backwards and forwards: which instrument to use, when to use them, when to worry about blood loss, when to work fast to get a depressed baby out, how to stop excessive bleeding, and on and on. We went over the procedure until I was satisfied she knew the answers and felt somewhat confident.

Three days later we had our first opportunity: Grace had prolonged labor with this first baby, no progress, and now there was early fetal distress—a perfect "first-case" for Sister Perpetua because there wouldn't be any adhesions from previous surgery. We prepared Grace for the O.R, and I said, "Are you ready for this?"

With her usual smile and a nervous giggle, she replied, "I guess so. Just so you're there to help me."

"I'll be there and you'll do fine."

She gave the spinal anesthetic. We scrubbed, dressed in sterile gowns and gloves, and placed the drapes. Standing on the right side and on her usual step stool, she took the scalpel, stopped to bow her head to say a "Hail Mary," and began. Her first cut was minuscule, with hardly a drop of blood. Her hands were shaking as she dabbed with a swab and made another tiny cut. I bit my tongue to not criticize, remembering my first C-section and how the teaching surgeon was so virtuously patient with me. Patience was not one of my strong suits, but I was determined not to hurry her. *Dear God, give me patience—and I need it now!* My impatience surged through, "Sister Perpetua, we'll never get through if you don't use more pressure to cut."

"I know."

'Use more force and get right through the skin and fat, down to the fascia.'

"Okay." She moved with a bit more alacrity and was soon opening the peritoneum.

"Bladder blade please," she said to me. I inserted it to give good exposure. With care, she made a small transverse incision in the lower uterus, inserted an index finger from each hand into the opening, and pulled it wide enough for the baby to come through. She put her hand under the head, gradually and gently delivering the head into the opening. I suctioned the baby's mouth while she delivered the rest of the baby—a beautiful girl. She clamped and cut the cord and handed the baby to Sister Rosemary. She asked for uterine clamps, used them to grab the edges of the uterine opening, and said, "Two 'O' chromic please." She methodically and competently—if rather slowly—closed the uterus in two layers. She needed help in tying knots—*we must work on knot tying, I see.* She had some problems correctly holding the needle holder—*we'll work on that too.* After closing the uterus, she suctioned and swabbed and checked for bleeding. Nothing significant. Then asked for a sponge count—*don't want to leave a sponge in the belly.* So far the operation had taken 70 minutes, not bad for a first C-section. I probably was way too antsy at times and I'm sure she knew it, but I would get better and so would she.

She was used to closing the abdomen, so now it was time for me to break scrub, check out the crying baby, and say, "Makorokoto (congratulations) Sister Perpetua. Your first C-section. Good Job." Everyone in the O.R. clapped and echoed, "Makorokoto Sister Perpetua."

She shyly looked around and answered, "Masvita (thank you)."

Over the next three months, I assisted as she did five more sections, some of them difficult cases. She learned what to do and what not to do, how to stay out of trouble and how to control bleeding, but most of all she learned how to be confident.

Difficult times require different solutions. During the next five years, there was no doctor at Silveira for most of the time because of the war. A Red Cross doctor flew in once a month, but of course he was never there when a C-section was needed. Sister Perpetua did twenty sections during the five years.

Makorokoto, Sister Perpetua.

Letter from Loretta: *November 30, 1975*

Dear Mom and Dad,

Glad to hear that you are out of the hospital and doing well Dad. I'm sure you both will be glad to get home. The time is getting close for us to go now, three and a half weeks. Dick has most of his preparing done, and I am just ready to start mine. There is not so much, as our big shipment has been sent. We leave the 17th. Our flight leaves at 2:00 p .m. and arrives in London at 8:00 a.m. We stay at a hotel near the airport overnight, and leave the next day at 2:00p.m., arriving in Chicago at 5:30 p.m., but we cross 4 or 5 time zones, so it is longer than it looks. Then we fly to Green Bay, and from there by car to Shawano. Donna and John have rented a four bedroom, furnished house about 6 miles out of town on the lake. It is a summer home for a doctor from Chicago, and we have to be out by May.

We've had a busy week. Monday I took the children to school, and brought the three little ones along so we could buy traveling clothes. They behaved well 'till about 11:00 o'clock, and then I had to keep after them all the time. It was really tiring. We picked up Mary and Doug after school to get their clothes, and were successful in finding something for everyone, even me, so tired and grumpy. We started home at half past four, arriving in time for supper.

Last week, Dick and I went in to Salisbury. Dick had an Association of Rhodesian Christian Hospitals meeting on Thursday, and had some other business to get done. We had dinner with friends, the Johnson's, an American couple who are Methodist Missionaries. The meeting was to be at their home the next day, and when Dick arrived for the meeting, they were just bundling Gene off to the hospital to have his appendix out. He is such a nut, when he filled out the hospital forms, in the space after sex he put semi-annually. They held the meeting anyway, and it went very well.

So did Gene's operation. We went to see him next day, and he was sitting on the side of the bed, swinging his feet like a kid. He's a Grandfather.

We stayed Thursday and Friday with the Davies family, and went to a play on Friday night. It wasn't very good, but it was nice to get dressed up and have my hair done anyway. Saturday we came home, stopping at Driefontein for lunch with the Brown's, and picked up Mike and Tom. Tom won a prize for a short story. It was really well done.

Sunday was the Ordination of one of our African priests. There were over 4 thousand people here. It was really a colorful sight, and an interesting experience. Drumming all night for two nights, dancing all day, and it was so hot. There were people from all the missions, so we said lots of "goodbyes" to so many good friends.

Today I have to get ready for Mr. Swainson from OXFAM, the organization that finances Dick's malnutrition work. He's a nice guy, and we will enjoy the visit, but we're are a bit tired of socializing. Well, I had better get Paul and begin his schoolwork. I'm going to have to quit that soon. Things are piling up.

Bye for now, hope you had a nice Thanksgiving.

Love and God bless,

Loretta

DRAFTED

Week before Thanksgiving, 18 November 1975:

An official registered letter arrived from the Rhodesian Government. With trepidation I opened it and read:

To: Richard Stoughton, M.D.

Silveira Hospital

Bikita District

Rhodesia

From: Department of Rhodesian Army

Salisbury, Rhodesia.

Subject: Reporting for physical exam for draft.

Sir:

You are directed to proceed to the Fort Victoria Army Depot for a physical exam on Wednesday, 10 December 1975 at 10:00 A.M.

All Foreign Nationals who have resided in Rhodesia longer than three years are subject to being drafted into the Rhodesian Army.

Signed,

_____

Oh my God. Now what do I do? I ran down to Father Kilchmann's office. He was the Superior for the mission with years of experience in Rhodesia, and loads of knowledge of the workings of the white government. After reading the letter, he looked up at me and said, "Yes, I heard they were going to do this, but didn't think it would be so soon. It seems the civil war isn't going well. They need more soldiers, especially in the medical field."

"I haven't heard of an increase in the war. What have you heard?"

"Activity's increasing, especially in the border areas. The Blacks are determined to have majority rule, and they don't want to wait."

"I understand, but not with violence. I hoped they'd work it out through the political system."

"The Rhodesian Government gives 'too little too late' for any real progress, so guerilla warfare is where it's going."

"Is there danger here at Silveira? Should I be worried about my family? What about our kids at boarding school?"

"I think it's safe for now."

"What about the new doctor that's coming in March?"

"I don't expect the activity to move away from the border areas anytime soon. The Rhodesian Army is too strong for that. If things should change, we'll be sure he and his family are safe."

"What about you being drafted? You've been here for ages."

"No, we religious are exempted. Too bad we can't suddenly make you one of our Brothers."

"What should I do? I could lose U.S. citizenship for being in a foreign army. I don't want to serve in their dirty war. I won't!"

"Go to the District Commissioner in Bikita. Perhaps he can help you."

Early Monday I drove the eight miles over the rough road to Bikita. Mr. Baker-Brown, the District Commissioner, was friendly but he toed the Rhodesian Front party line of "white rule forever."

After showing him the letter, I said, "You know I'm the only doctor for the 80,000 people in Bikita District. What am I to do?"

"Go for the physical, and then wait and see. Maybe you'll be lucky and not be called up."

"I could lose my U.S. citizenship if I serve in a foreign army."

"That's not our concern. The law says you're eligible for the draft. The only exemptions are for religious, or people with disabilities, or over the age of fifty."

"What if I refuse?"

"You'll be put in jail."

"There's no way to get out of this?"

"Afraid not."

My replacement from Mission Doctors Association in Los Angeles wasn't due to arrive until March or April. I wanted to be there to welcome him, introduce him to the work, and hope that all the outreach activities would be continued. Now everything would have to change. I couldn't stay and take the risk of being drafted into the Rhodesian Army.

The next four weeks were a blur. I went to Fort Victoria to send a telegram to Mission Doctors Association, explaining the situation in as few words as possible, and requesting them to arrange a flight for us from Salisbury to Green Bay, Wisconsin, preferably just before Christmas. I sent another telegram to my sister Donna in Shawano, Wisconsin saying we would be arriving in late December. Could they please find a place for us to live? Finally, another to my contact at the Clinic stating I hoped to start working January 2nd if that was o.k. Brother Serafin made some wooden crates for shipping our "valuables" home and we packed what would fit. By December

17th, everything was ready for us to leave Silveira early the next morning, drive to Salisbury and leave on the noon flight to London, then to Chicago, and finally to Green Bay.

Of course, we couldn't leave without a "farewell party" for the Stoughton Family. Even though our possessions were packed, I received a final gift: an African beaded necklace that had multiple circular wooden plaques with inscriptions: *Multipurpose Dispenser of TLC; Sprinter King; Arch-enemy of Slipped Ligatures; Perpetual Mobile; Life President of C.S.P. (Common Sense People); Conqueror of Malnutrition; Air Chief Marshal of Chipungu Fleet;* and my favorite, *Jack of All Trades.* I still have it hanging in my living room.

It was a wonderful party, both celebratory and sad, breaking up at 11:00. I drank my limit of three beers and we headed home to bed. I was barely asleep when for one last time there was that loud banging on the door, "Doctor, come quick. There's been an accident and several men are injured."

Oh no, can't I even have one last night of uninterrupted sleep? Barely able to navigate in the dark down the steps and up the hill, I arrived to find several of the Sisters sorting out injuries from a car accident. Men who were working on the power line to bring electricity to the mission had been out partying. I know I had beer on my breath, but they smelled like a brewery, and acted like they'd been drinking for hours.

Five men injured. *Dick, turn on your "auto-pilot."* You quickly triage to see who's most serious. All are moaning and groaning, so nothing life-threatening, at least not yet. You give orders to get a blood pressure and pulse on each one. You methodically move from one to the next. First one: chest is clear; abdomen soft; eyes normal; moves all extremities; lacerations and abrasions on both arms; you tell Sister Rita to sew this one up and clean his abrasions. Next: obvious broken arm but position looks good. Get an x-ray in the morning; put on a splint tonight. Next: only abrasions on both arms; you tell a student nurse to clean the abrasions and put on a clean dressing.

Next: another obvious broken arm, but this will need setting; you tell Sister Amoris to take an x-ray right away so you can fix it. Next: no injuries obvious; maybe some bruises on his back, but nothing serious. You write quick orders on each and have them all admitted to the male ward. The man is back from x-ray; both bones broken at the wrist and slightly displaced; you give just a bit of morphine for pain—he doesn't need much because of an abundance of alcohol floating around—you give a good pull on the hand and wrist, set the fracture, place a plaster splint on both sides of the wrist and wrap it with an ace bandage; you order an x-ray for the morning. It's 3:00 A.M. as you slowly make your way home to a warm bed, one last time looking up at the bright stars of the Southern Hemisphere, thinking, *Can't leave without one last Hurrah. It's a wonder there wasn't a C-section.*

Early the morning of the December 18, 1975 the nine of us piled into the VW Combi Van while another vehicle followed with our pile of luggage. We said our tearful goodbyes to everyone and were off. Two miles from the mission, in the rearview mirror I had my last vision of the mission sitting at the base of the mountain. I said another silent *Goodbye Silveira*. We arrived at the airport just in time to make our flight. With a mountain of luggage in front of the terminal—18 checked bags and one carry-on for each—we had a final picture taken of the Stoughton Clan in Rhodesia.

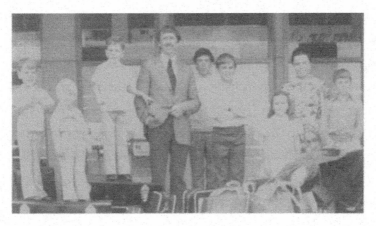

Ready to leave, L-R: Paul, Tim, Pete, Dick, Mike, Tom, Mary, Loretta, Doug

Walking into the terminal we frantically looked for Mary's shoes. She was always barefoot at the mission, so thought nothing of removing them for the picture. We looked everywhere, no success. Time to leave. As we walked through customs, Mary held up a shoe on each hand to show them to Sister Rosemary. Waving a final goodbye, we boarded the British Airways plane to London.

As it gained altitude, I looked out the window and wondered, *Will we ever come back? What lies in store for us now? How will we cope with life in the U.S.? I'm used to being alone and 'in charge.' Now I'll be one of nine in a clinic, and the junior doctor, even though I'm 38. How's that going to work? Will I fit in? How will Loretta and the kids do? We're going from the heat of summer to the cold of winter in Wisconsin. Hope they have some warm clothes for us. . . .* and I dozed off to dream of Silveira: The white church in the middle, our house on the hill to the left, the hospital on the opposite hill to the right. The hordes of patients, the wonderful people, the busy days, zzzzzzzzzz.

*

Our trip to Green Bay was not without complications. With our luggage checked through to Chicago, we stayed overnight in a hotel in London near the airport. Getting all nine of us up in time for an early morning flight wasn't easy, but we made it, and were on our way to Chicago. We had three hours between flights in Chicago, thinking that would be plenty of time. However, the baggage handlers were having a "slowdown" protest, so all the luggage came up the belt one bag at a time with several minutes or more between each bag. Everyone in the area was impatient, our kids were getting wild, and tempers were flaring. After 90 minutes, I began worrying about making the flight to Green Bay. A very large and friendly African American customs agent came over with a smile on his face, looked at our pile of luggage and all the kids and said, "Let me know when you have everything and I'll get you right through." *Thank you God.*

My Aunt Ethel was standing behind the waiting-area glass waving at us and hoping she could spend some time with us between flights. When we finally had our luggage there was only time for a quick hug, and we had to hurry to the main terminal. *Dear God, how do we get there with all this stuff?* A large van outside the International Terminal was waiting for someone who hadn't arrived, and the driver offered to take us to the main terminal. *Thank you God.* With 30 minutes to catch our flight, I hurried to the front of the line at check-in, explained our problem, paid $50 for an oversized bag, hurried through the terminal to our gate, and boarded just as the doors were closing. *Thanks again God.*

We landed in Green Bay in a blowing snowstorm. Stepping off the plane, Tom, with a grin on his face said, "Gee, it seems like just yesterday it was summer!"

My sister and her husband and friends greeted us. In several cars they drove us through the blowing snow to our temporary home on the shores of frozen Shawano Lake. We awoke the next morning to the sound of a snow-blower clearing a foot of fresh snow from our driveway.

EPILOGUE TO PART ONE

For the next 26 years we lived a very average "small-town-Midwest" lifestyle in Shawano, Wisconsin. In Rhodesia, things were far from normal. Missionaries provided 90% of educational and medical services in rural Rhodesia, but this didn't exempt them from the violence unleashed by the black guerilla warriors between 1976 and 1980. Many missionaries were brutally raped and killed. Silveira had "visits" from the terrorists, but fortunately no killings or other atrocities. Father Kilchmann remained determinedly "neutral," dealing with the men in a firm but compassionate manner. He believed in their goals but not their methods. Student nurses and boys from the Secondary School were forced to attend "educational meetings" up the mountain. Some of the nurses, after being indoctrinated into their ideology, decided to join them, becoming girlfriends or "wives" of the leaders. In late 1976, because of the increasing danger, my replacement and his family were forced to leave, going to a mission in Malawi. Finally, in 1980 a political agreement was forged and Black Independence was declared, with Robert Mugabe being elected as the first leader of the newly named Zimbabwe. He remained in that position until November, 2019 when he was replaced by Emmerson Mnangagwa in what has been called a "non-coup" coup. Mugabe and Mnanagagwa have both proven to be brutal and corrupt plutocrats.

PROLOGUE FOR PART TWO:

Summer 2000, Chambers Island, in the
Green Bay waters of Lake Michigan:

" . . . We cannot do everything, and there is a sense of liberation in realizing that. This enables us to do something and to do it very well. It may be incomplete, but it is a beginning, a step along the way, an opportunity for the Lord's Grace to enter and do the rest." [3]

As we walked along the bluff overlooking the blue, cold water of Lake Michigan, gulls swooped over the coastline, raucously cawing at each other while waves from the previous nights' storm pounded noisily upon the rocky shore. Bishop Robert Morneau, our retreat-master, had just handed us the "Romero Prayer," part of which is above. The theme of the retreat was "Service." His sermon was concise: "We are all called to give service back to God. What is He calling you to do *today*?"

Loretta and I walked away from the Retreat Center so we could keep the silence of the area but still talk about the message—we both felt it was aimed directly at us. Loretta said, "Dick, maybe we've been selfish in thinking we can't do long-term missionary work after you retire. Our kids have stable marriages and are doing well. They don't need us around to tell them what to do. I think we should go back to Zimbabwe for longer than just a few months. What do you think?"

---

3   From "The Romero Prayer." Popularized because Archbishop Romero was martyred in El Salvador shortly after giving this prayer to a group of priests at a retreat. It was actually composed by Bishop Ken Untener of Saginaw, Michigan, and drafted for a homily by Cardinal John Dearden in Nov. 1979 for a celebration of departed priests. Because of the popularity of Archbishop Romero, it has mistakenly been labeled, "The Romero Prayer."

I was planning to retire from my busy medical practice in Shawano, Wisconsin the next year, and we were struggling with what to do to give meaning to our lives after retirement. We discussed many options: short-term missionary work; one to two month relief stints on Indian Reservations; Cruise Ship Doctor; or just retire and play golf as much as possible. The last two were quickly discarded as "not for us." Because of our previous work in Rhodesia in the 1970's, any type of missionary work was attractive.

I replied, "That's exactly what I think. I'd love to go back to Zimbabwe. Let's talk it over with Bishop Morneau." I immediately knew this was a call we could not ignore. By noon, I had a "to do list" with 20 items on it—what we would have "to do" to make it happen: clean out the basement and attic; give away furniture to the kids; put the house up for sale; start studying about the treatment of AIDS in Africa; update our immunizations; arrange for someone to manage my IRA's; and on and on. Even now, it's amazing when I think how easy it was that everything fell so quickly into place. Likewise the discussion with our seven kids: "We knew you were going to do that," they replied. *We* didn't know it until that day on Chambers Island, but they did. So began another *Step Along the Way* for us to return to Zimbabwe for eight more years working at a rural Mission Hospital.

"Romero Prayer"

It helps, now and then, to step back and take the long view. The Kingdom is not only beyond our efforts, it is even beyond our vision. We accomplish in our lifetime only a tiny fraction of the magnificent enterprise that is the Lord's work. Nothing we do is complete, which is another way of saying that the Kingdom always lies beyond us.

No statement says all that should be said. No prayer fully expresses our faith. No confession brings perfection, no pastoral visit brings wholeness. No program accomplished the Church's mission. No set of goals and objectives includes everything.

This is what we are about. We plant the seeds that one day will grow. We water seeds already planted, knowing that they will need further development. We provide yeast that produces effects far beyond our capabilities.

We cannot do everything and there is a sense of liberation in realizing that. This enables us to do *something*, and to do it very well. It may be incomplete, but it is a beginning, a step along the way, an opportunity for the Lord's Grace to enter and do the rest. We may never see the end results, but that is the difference between the master builder and the worker. We are workers, not master builders, ministers, not messiahs. We are prophets of a future that is not our own.

RE-ENTRY

September 2001: Our return to mission life in Zimbabwe was supposed to start with a golf vacation in Ireland with friends from Wisconsin, leaving Chicago on September 12, 2001. On the 11th, Doug (our thirdborn) and I were driving through a Chicago suburb looking for last-minute computer items when we heard the news: *An airplane has hit the World Trade Center.*

We immediately returned to Doug's house and sat mesmerized as a second plane hit the other tower with a horrifying surge of smoke and debris blasting out the opposite side as if the plane flew straight through the building. Then a plane hitting the Pentagon, leaving an ugly black smoldering hole; another plane heading for D.C. but went off the radar in Pennsylvania. Through splayed fingers, we watched people jump from upper floors of the twin towers to certain death, and sat in silence as both structures collapsed as if in slow motion. Hordes of people on the streets of New York were running through the canyons of buildings, desperately trying to escape the blast of dirt, debris, and black smoke that was roiling down the corridors of Manhattan like some horror movie, only this was real-time life in terrifying color. *Was the entire nation under terrorist attack?*

September 11th would live alongside Pearl Harbor as "twin days of infamy." We would forever be on the lookout for new terrorist activity. Does that backpack have a bomb in it? Does that man look suspicious? Paranoia ran amok. As we boarded airplanes in the future, we would expect and accept long check-in lines and delays as we meekly passed through security checkpoints. Everyone would remember where they were and what they were doing on 9-11.

The five-day delay for our trip was a mere inconvenience—nothing compared to the thousands of families whose lives were irrevocably devastated by the attacks. Because we had the tickets, on September 17th we still flew to Ireland by ourselves—the group vacation couldn't be rescheduled on short notice—and then to Switzerland and finally to Zimbabwe. We felt safe because security was the tightest we ever experienced before or since. It was supposed to be a joyful holiday before starting our new life, but there wasn't much joy—only sadness over the events of 9-11. We were pleasantly surprised and deeply appreciative of the outpouring of love shown by strangers we met as we travelled through Ireland: "I'm so sorry for what happened in the U.S.;" "You have our condolences;" "It's so sad. Who could be so evil?" — were just a few of the comments from the many people who specifically came up to us to express their sorrow and outrage. In Switzerland, we met old friends at the Bethlehem Fathers and Brothers Motherhouse, where more healing occurred, allowing us to depart for Zimbabwe in a spirit of love and friendship.

*

Arriving in Harare was surreal. So much had changed, and yet so much was still the same: New buildings and new roads and new majority rule, but the same old poverty, same amount of malnutrition, and too many people living on less than a dollar a day. In the years to come, I wouldn't see one case of measles or whooping cough, but the AIDS epidemic was scything down victims like so many wheat stalks in a defenseless field.

Many cities and towns had new names: Harare for Salisbury; Masvingo for Fort Victoria; Chivhu for Enkeldoorn; Zvishavane for Shabani; Gweru for Gwelo; and so on. We arrived at a relatively new and modern International Terminal, but indications of a faltering economy were apparent by the dim lights, stopped up toilets without tissue, and a baggage conveyor belt that refused to run. With toe-tapping impatience we waited for porters to carry our luggage from the plane to the terminal. Gruff customs agents stared us in the eye as if to say, "Why are you here? What does a white person want in our country?" By their actions we felt unwelcome. *I wonder if they treat all tourists this way or are they just having a bad day? No wonder tourism is down.* Perusing my passport, the agent asked me, "What is the purpose of your visit?"

Because I didn't yet have a license to practice medicine in the country, I answered, "Visiting old friends." I could work without a license as long as another doctor was at the hospital, and if we decided to return for long-term, I would pay $500 and apply for a renewal of the license I had in the 1970's.

"Where will you be staying?"

"With the Dominican Sisters at Fourth Street, and later at St. Theresa Hospital in Chirumanzu District."

"Do you have anything to declare?"

"No, I only have a few inexpensive gifts for some of the Sisters."

He looked at me, then at Loretta, then at our bags and back at me, frowned and said, "O.K. Next!"—and we were through customs and into the arrivals area, where Dominican Sisters Patricia and Rosemary were waiting with open arms. After hugs and kisses, we all began talking at once:

"It's so good to see you."

"We're glad to be here."

"You look just the same."

"You too."

"Except I'm a bit greyer."

"Aren't we all?"

"How was your flight and how are the children? Tell us all about them." Even though it had been 26 years, the Sisters still thought of our kids as the "children" they knew, even though our youngest was now twenty-eight.

We knew both of them from the '70's—Sister Rosemary was a close friend because she was with us at Silveira, even babysitting for us at times.

Sister Patricia visited us there in '74. She took our outreach programs and expanded and improved on them at St. Theresa Hospital, where we were now going for our "trial return to missionary life" for the next three months. Patricia was my contact person once we made the decision to return to Zimbabwe. She's a 5-foot 10-inch Irish Dominican Nun who is a ball of fire with a sharp Irish wit, and a font of information and contacts. Whenever I wanted to get a scarce item, I first went to her. If she didn't know where to get it, she knew someone who did. She became our lifeline and "go-to-person" for the next eight years.

Driving from the airport into the city was different from the 70's. A four-lane divided highway pointed directly to the city center, but it was no longer new, was pockmarked with deep potholes, garbage and loose papers littering the streets "Yes, there's no money for road repair these days," Sister Pat informed us as she weaved her way like someone evading road mines. "Right now, all the money is being used to keep the War Vets quiet. Political unrest within the ruling ZANU-PF party is rampant, especially among the vets of the war for independence. Mugabe keeps them quiet by paying them off." After 21 years as the leader of the country, 76-year-old Robert Mugabe was still firmly in control of the wheels of government. If he needed more funds, he told the Reserve Bank to "print more money and pay the war vets." Then, when that predictably resulted in inflation of 130%, he blamed it on sanctions imposed by U.S. President George Bush and U.K. Prime Minister Tony Blair. Little did we know that we would *yearn* for inflation of *only 130%* in the years ahead.

Driving through Harare we saw a different city from what we knew in the '70's. The main thoroughfare was still wide—wide enough to make a 180-degree turn with a six-span oxen team when the streets were laid out in the early 1900's—but new skyscrapers dotted the skyline. In Harare, anything over five stories was considered a "skyscraper." After Independence in 1980, money poured in from around the world, resulting in massive building projects, including several twenty to thirty-story buildings in Harare, plus a new and expanded road system throughout the country. Now the foreign money had dried up, tax revenues were falling, and the country couldn't afford the upkeep. The results were apparent as we bumped through the streets of this once impressive city: inoperative traffic lights, deep potholes, garbage littering the streets and alleyways, dilapidated busses belching black smoke, and a multitude of street vendors at every stoplight trying to eke out an existence by selling phone cards, cigarettes, newspapers, and odds and ends.

The social fabric of the country was slowly but inexorably crumbling because the glue that held it together, the highly successful but mostly white-owned commercial farms, were illegally being taken over by inexperienced blacks with little or no agricultural expertise. There was a need to solve the land inequity problem, but Mugabe's butcher-hatchet method wasn't the answer. You've heard the saying, "He cut off his nose to spite his face?" Mugabe did just that when he became angry with the white farmers because of a vote that went against him in 2000 on a new constitution. When that referendum was defeated, Mugabe decided to throw the White farmers off their farms "to show them who was in power." Many of the newly anointed black farmers knew little about the hard work and science required for successful farming. Many were higher-up bureaucrats with no desire to farm—they only wanted to sell the ill-gotten tractors and other farm equipment, live in a nice house on weekends, and act like "land barons," without putting any effort into growing the agriculture products the country so desperately needed. During the next eight years we painfully watched this once beautiful agricultural country sink into a morass of inefficiency, with huge areas of previously productive farmland lying fallow. Factories related to the farm economy went bankrupt, unemployment soared to over 90%, annual inflation of over 100% became "normal," and the economy spiraled downward. A country that once enjoyed the epithet of being "The Breadbasket of Southern Africa" could no longer grow enough food for its own people.

As we drove through Harare, I noticed not only the new buildings, but also the lack of white faces. *Where have all the white people gone? When we were here in the '70's, Salisbury was filled with white faces. Now there are so few. Have they been forced out?*

The Sisters drove us to Emerald Hill, one of their establishments in a suburb of Harare. Situated on 100 acres on top of a hill, it consisted of a small church and convent, an orphanage for 100 children, and a large Boarding School for the Deaf. A small apartment complex near the church and next to the orphanage became our "home away from home" when we visited Harare. It suited our purposes because the complex was fenced and guarded—providing us with a degree of security—and we could come and go without interfering with others, but still be part of the community when we wanted. Yes, safety had become a big issue during the intervening 26 years. Most homes in Harare that once showcased beautiful yards and gardens visible from the street were now surrounded with tall cement walls topped with razor wire, an armed guard at the gate. In many parts of the world people are withdrawing into their own personal bunkers and losing a piece of their humanity in the process. Neighbors no longer are "the Jones's next door," but are "those people on the other side of the wall who we only glimpse as they drive through their security gate." I've never been a "city person" and don't like spending much time in cities, so I was glad we would be living in a totally open environment at St. Theresa's.

That evening we had supper with several of the Sisters, with many new and old faces—always a problem for me who has so much trouble remembering faces and names, a kind of "face blindness" to go along with my color blindness. It was embarrassing when I would have to ask one of the African Sisters her name, and she would say, "But Doctor Stoughton, don't you remember me?"

That Sunday, all 100 orphans plus many of the surrounding area Catholics attended Mass at Emerald Hill. The small church was packed and there was an electric excitement in the air. Through the open windows we could hear the birds singing as if they wanted to be part of the celebration.

A fresh breeze brought the pleasant odor of Jacaranda blossoms as subdued whispering awaited the beginning of Mass. Older orphans read the first and second readings, in their slightly Shona-ized English—a kind of sing-songy English that was pleasant to hear but difficult for my hearing-impaired ears to discern. High-pitched singing voices accompanied by guitars and drums filled the church to introduce the Gospel, and then came the homily by 80-year-old Jesuit Father Patrick Maloney. Loretta leaned my way and whispered, "*This* is where we're supposed to be and isn't it good to be back?"

The next day, Sister Rosemary drove us to St. Theresa's, a drive of 120 miles on a fairly good blacktop road (dodging the ever present potholes) and then 20 miles on a terrible sandy and rough road. We stopped at the post office in Mvuma (it was Umvuma when our boys went to school there in 1970) to get mail for the hospital—a necessity whenever anyone was near the small town. After stopping for a coke, I told Sister Rosemary I would like to drive so I could once again get used to driving "on the wrong side of the road." Going up a small hill just out of Mvuma, I nearly hit a large male Kudu with a beautiful rack of spiral horns as he bounded across the road. Sister Rosemary said, "Stop. There's usually more than one."

After stopping, we looked to the left to see three young males standing very still and staring at us—a perfect photo-op with my telephoto lens. Sister Rosemary whispered, "You know, they're welcoming you back to Zimbabwe."

A few miles later, we turned onto the dirt road and I saw it was going to be a challenge. Twists and turns, ups and downs, and in some areas I wondered if we were on the road or out in a field. At one river crossing, a steep embankment with deep ruts cutting through the road made it difficult to decide which was the best path down to the bridge. Sister Rosemary said, "Stay on the right. This was nearly impassable a few weeks ago when the river was in flood." *Was impassable? Looks to me like it is now.*

With the car in first gear, I slowly inched my way down the steep hill, leaning sharply to the right and then to the left and finally bouncing onto the cement bridge. "Whew, hope that's the worst," I said.

'Oh, it is," laughed Rosemary.

We passed several villages that looked the same as in the 70's, except now there were a few square shaped cement-block houses in addition to the traditional round huts with grass-thatched roofs. Fields were being prepared for planting, with men walking behind oxen-pulled plows, their young boys running ahead and beating the ox with a stick to keep it moving. *This is 21st Century farming?* The rock strewn sandy fields didn't look like they would support much agriculture, and they didn't. In a good year, a farmer might get 20 bushels of maize per acre—in the U.S. the average is over 140. In a bad year, they might get nothing, and historically three out of five years were bad. Such was the lot of a subsistence farmer, with many not growing enough food for their own family. Twenty-one years after Independence and the lot of the poor rural farmer was unchanged. The take-over of white-owned farms would not improve the situation. A white minority aristocracy was replaced by a black majority autocracy, and the poor continued to suffer.

*

Introduction to the hospital and mission was a flurry of activity and confusion: a new house to live in; more new faces and names; new schedules; and most daunting of all was the disease of AIDS. It would dominate my thought processes for the next eight years. St. Theresa Hospital had a bed capacity of 165 patients, and when we arrived it was nearly full, with 70% of the non-obstetric beds being AIDS patients with varying opportunistic infections: tuberculosis, fungal and bacterial meningitis, heart infections, pneumonias, diarrheas, skin infections, skin cancers, and most with severe wasting—the reason AIDS is called "Slim Disease." Some of the infections were treatable and some weren't. The best I could hope for was to get each patient well enough to go home for a few more months of a miserable existence. In Zimbabwe there was no treatment for the AIDS virus; no hope for long-term recovery; no hope—only despair for men and women and children and infants. Every family was affected by the AIDS pandemic. One of the African Sisters told me that at a relatives' funeral, she and her cousins sat around to reminisce and count the number of relatives that had died of AIDS during the past decade—they counted fifty-five deaths in that one large extended family.

Twenty-five percent of Zimbabweans between the age of 18 and 50 were HIV positive and were dying at a rate of 3,000 per week—more than 150,000 a year in this country of 12 million. To put it into perspective: one night shortly after we arrived, there was a terrible accident. A bus hit a large truck head on, instantly killing 30 young college students. It received international news coverage. People were devastated by the sudden deaths of so many young people. And yet, AIDS was causing the equivalent of 100 bus accidents *every week of the year!* In a time of high unemployment, coffin making was a thriving business. *I thought measles and whooping cough was bad? There's none of those cases now, but AIDS is worse by a magnitude of 100. How can I possibly make a difference? Am I called to do this work just to give Hospice care to the dying? Then I remembered the Romero Prayer: ". . . We cannot do everything, and there is a sense of liberation in realizing that, because it allows us to do something and to do it very well." I needed to start doing "something."*

*

Three weeks after our arrival, we returned to Harare on hospital business. While there, Loretta wanted to shop for supplies for our house, so on a Saturday morning we went to a modern shopping center in one of the suburbs. After scouring the stores, there was still one item she needed and asked me to drive into the city center so she could shop at Meikles, a well-known department store. Because the car was nearly out of diesel, I dropped her at the front entrance and told her I would be back as soon as I filled the car. Fifteen minutes later I returned to find the store closed—we hadn't realized that all stores closed at 1:00 PM on Saturdays. She was nowhere to be seen and there were hordes of black people rushing to the bus depot. I've never thought of myself as racist nor even of being "race conscious," but that day I was very aware that I was the only white person driving around and I was worried because I didn't see the one white face I so much wanted to see. *Where could she be? Has something happened to her? Has she been assaulted by some of these rough-looking men? Where is she?*

Neither of us had a cell phone, so all I could do was keep driving around the block, hoping to catch sight of that one white face. No luck. I drove the eight blocks to the Dominican Convent on Fourth Street. No luck. Back to Meikles. Nothing. Back to Fourth street where I asked the guard to call Sister Patricia. She came to the entrance, I told her my concerns, and together we drove around and around the downtown area as she tried to reassure me Loretta was alright, but we couldn't find her and I was becoming even more worried and anxious.

She called a number she had been given to use "in case of emergency." Soon a black man in a nice suit arrived, and Sister introduced me to Patrick Ngoma. I later learned he was with the CIO (Central Intelligence—like our CIA, or maybe I should say the KGB?) and that he was an infamous "war vet" who was rumored to be mean and dangerous. Not that day—he was most accommodating and helpful. He told me, "We haven't had any cases of white tourists being assaulted, so I'm sure she's alright. She must have gone some place where she felt safe. Where might that be?"

"We already checked at the Fourth Street Convent, and I can't get any-one to answer a phone at Emerald Hill, but that's five miles away, so I doubt she would have gone there," answered Sister Patricia.

Together we drove around with no success. With each passing moment, my worry increased. "What more can we do?" I asked.

Sister Patricia said to Patrick, "Could she have been picked up by a policeman and taken to the police station?"

"I don't think so," answered Patrick. "But let's go and see."

Just as we walked up the stairs to the police station, Patricia's cell phone rang, with the news that Loretta was sitting on the steps of the apartment at Emerald Hill. My eyes fill with tears of joy.

Because Patrick had been so helpful, Patricia invited him back to the Convent for a cold coke and he accepted. She could see how antsy I was, so she turned to me and said, "Why don't you go back to Emerald Hill and see how Loretta is?"

Arriving there, I gave her a quick hug and told her how helpless I felt. "Why did you come all the way back here and not go to the Fourth Street Convent? I was so worried. I didn't know what to do."

"We're staying here, so I thought it would be the logical place to go. When I found the store was closed and so many black people swarming about and not one white face, I was scared. I grabbed a taxi and the only thing I could think of was to have him bring me here. I'm sorry, but I didn't know what else to do."

"I just wish you'd gone to Fourth Street, 'cause then I would have found you right away."

"Sorry, to me it seemed the logical thing."

*

It gave me a new perspective on my concept of "race." I really hadn't thought much about it before. When we were in Rhodesia in the 70's, we lived and worked with predominantly black people and never felt out of place or overwhelmed or unsafe. When we shopped in Fort Victoria or Salisbury, there were many white people mixed in with the blacks, so I never felt like a minority. In the U.S. we lived in predominantly white communities. Now when I walked down the streets of Harare and only saw an occasional white face, it bothered me. Why? It bothered me, and I was bothered by the fact that it bothered me. Does that make sense? I realized how easily I ascribed evil intentions to those black people near Meikles just because "they looked different." Would I have felt the same if they had been white? Probably not.

*

Just as we were ready to leave for St. Theresa's that Sunday, Sister Gabriel asked me to look at a young boy in the orphanage who had a deep burn on his right forearm. Gift was a three-year-old boy who lived with his grandmother in a shantytown North of Harare. One evening his sweater caught fire, burning his right forearm. Sister Patricia saw the burn while working at their weekly medical clinic in the shantytown. She knew it needed daily treatment, so she brought Gift back to the orphanage for Sister Gabriel to care for him until the burn healed.

Kneeling down and looking Gift in the eye, I said, "Can I look at this?" He didn't speak any English and I didn't speak much Shona, so Sister interpreted. He slowly nodded his head yes. He winced a bit as I took off the last of the bandages. There was a deep burn on his right forearm. "This is probably going to need a skin graft," I said to Sister.

"Oh, no. Now what am I going to do? He can't afford it and neither can we."

"I guess we could take him to St. Theresa's. I could put him on the pediatric ward, clean it up, and do a graft when it's clean." So, with no authorization other than Sister Gabriel saying it was okay, we took Gift with us. As we approached the Mission I started thinking about the children's ward, and how each child had a relative to look after them. I turned to Loretta and said, "Maybe we're going to have to take care of this boy until he's better. I don't think it'll work very well if he's alone on the children's ward."

"We can do that," she said, easily accepting this child into our house, as a mother of eight is likely to do. It worked fine until an unexpected telephone call from the U.S. came to the hospital—quite a miracle in itself since the phone seldom worked. It was Loretta's sister Barb with news that her husband had suddenly died of a heart attack. Loretta and Barb were very close, so we quickly made plans for Loretta to fly back to South Dakota for the funeral and spend some time with Barb afterwards. Now I was going to be an "old, single working Dad with a small child"—and a child that didn't speak English. Mai Wei—Woe is me.

The two of us developed a good routine: Monica, our maid, came at 8:00 AM and looked after Gift during the day; she brought him to the minor surgery for dressing change each day, fixed our noon meal, and stayed until I was home at 5:00. Then it was up to me until 8:00 the next morning. One day when I came home, Gift was still napping when Monica left. When he awoke, he started crying, with crocodile tears streaming down his face. What could I do? I held him and tried to soothe him, but nothing worked. I walked around the house tightly holding the weeping boy, but he continued to cry, so I thought he must be hungry. Sitting him on a chair in the kitchen, I fixed us something to eat, including a nice piece of meat, a special treat for the poorest Africans. I thought this would get his attention, but the sobbing persisted and he refused to eat. I slowly ate my meal and offered him small bites of meat, but he shook his head and kept on crying, shoulders shaking and tears flowing. I felt so sorry for this bereft little boy who didn't understand my English, but I didn't know what more to do. When I finished eating, he was still sobbing and his food was untouched. Not knowing what else to do, I picked up my plate, put it in the sink and then started to pick up his plate. He looked at me in alarm, grabbed the plate and set it down, quit crying, and gobbled down his food. End of crying jag, and once again the happy boy I had come to know and love.

Later that evening, I was sitting on the couch with him next to me, reading a children's book about hippos and crocodiles. After finishing the story, he continued looking at the pictures while I was working on my laptop. The transformer for the cord was sitting near him and he picked it up, held it to his ear, and said, "Moroi (Hello)." Pause. Then "Makidii (How are you?)." Pause. Then "Bye Bye," and placed the transformer down like he was hanging up a phone, and laughed and laughed. He repeated it over and over, laughing each time. His laugh was infectious and soon both of us were playing his silly telephone game with my computer transformer, with me answering him, and he ending with "Bye, Bye" and laughing.

In two weeks time his arm had healed without a skin graft. One of the Sisters was going to Harare so she took him back to the orphanage. The house felt empty and I was lonely.

The saga of Gift continued for some time. By the time we returned in 2002, the Sisters had discovered that he wasn't an orphan after all. The woman Sister Patricia watched being buried wasn't his mother, but his grandmother. His mother was only 14 when he was born, and the grandmother who died of AIDS was raising him. After she died, Gift was shuffled up the line to the great-grandmother.

We visited them at the shantytown several times. Even though we spent many years in Africa, we had never seen anything like this. Several miles North of the city, it was located in a large field, two hundred acres of rolling hills covered with all types of temporary and not-so-temporary shacks—heavy duty plastic cubicles with a few scraps of wood holding them together, some flimsy wooden structures, and here and there a small cement block building with asbestos sheeting on the roof. Some people had only a piece of plastic they pulled over themselves at night, and otherwise were in the open. A conservative estimate was 25,000 poor souls living in this shantytown called "Hatcliff Extension." Makeshift muddy roads wound through the area, and we saw long lines of youngsters working long-handled pumps to get safe water from the deep wells that were placed here and there by charitable organizations. Temporary shops were selling Coca-Cola, Fanta Orange, Chibuku beer (similar to "home-brew" and not requiring refrigeration), cell-phone cards, groceries, and other commodities. *Free enterprise finds a way to make money in any environment.*

When visiting Gift, we would take a few items of food and clothing and sweets, and we struggled to think of a way we might salvage this one child's life. He was obviously very smart and maybe we could do something? Even though we were warned to not get emotionally involved, we already were and Gift was special to us. We thought we might have a solution, so on one of our visits—through an interpreter—I said, "Ambuya, would you like to come with Gift to St. Theresa's and live there? We would find a nice place for you to live and find work for you at the hospital. Gift could go to the Mission school and we would pay his fees. What do you think?"

She poked in the fire, walked around, poked in the fire some more, hummed to herself, and finally said, "Come back tomorrow and I'll let you know."

The next day she agreed to come for a couple of months to see if she liked it. In the meantime we learned that Gift's mother was alive, but not interested in taking care of him. We had legal advice that *if* Gift started living at St. Theresa's with the great-grandmother, we needed a legal document stating she was his legal guardian so the mother wouldn't come demanding compensation and accusing us of kidnapping the boy. So on another trip to Harare we visited the now 17-year-old mother who was living in a crowded house in Chitingwisa—a huge overly crowded city just 20 miles South of Harare. She was living with a new boyfriend who had no desire to have a three-year-old as his responsibility. She readily signed our papers and we thought we had a good solution for Gift.

Not so fast. After three weeks, the Ambuya came and wanted to talk to us. With Monica as interpreter, she said, "I want to go back to Hatfield."

"I thought you agreed to stay for two months and then decide," I replied.

"It's too quiet here. I like the excitement of Hatfield. All my friends are there."

"What about Gift going to school?"

"I'll find a way to send him to school."

"How?"

'I don't know. The Sisters will help me. They always have."

When the next car went to Harare, Gift and the Ambuya were in the back and heading back to shantytown. She decided St. Theresa's was too "rural" and there wasn't enough excitement—even though there was a regular supply of food and firewood, she had a job, Gift could go to school, there was no danger, and it was the only hope for a good future for Gift. The pull of the shantytown was too great, so they left. I never understood it. *What pulls rural people into shantytowns all over the world? They go hoping for a better life, but when it's worse than what they had, they still don't want to return to their rural home. Maybe they don't want to admit failure? Maybe they really do like the excitement and danger? It seems they soon become ensconced citizens of a shantytown, and before they know it, they have established a second-generation family that doesn't know any other life.*

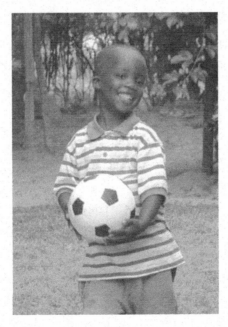

Gift

We continued to visit them when we were in Harare, taking the usual food and treats and used clothing. Gift was attending the pre-school run by the Dominican Sisters and seemed to be thriving. He had the nicest smile for us when we visited. Then in 2005, Mugabe and his thugs, in a grand scheme called Murambitsvina—meaning "Clean Up the Trash"— destroyed that shantytown and several others, uprooting upwards of 700,000 people in the process. With just one day of warning, bulldozers leveled the many acres of tarpaper shanties and wooden houses and cement block houses, with no place for the people to go. No planning—just "clean up the trash"—and the Hell with the people and the consequences. Elected officials—elected by some of those very same people they were displacing—decided the poor were unimportant when cleaning up the "trash of the shantytown." It was just one more hastily conceived plan by bureaucrats who had no concern for the poor. Maybe someone high up in government wanted the land and damn the people who got in the way? I don't know, but I do know that many died of exposure that winter. Everyone living in Hatfield Extension was displaced and we lost track of Gift. He would be in his 20's by now, and *if* he's alive, he's probably barely surviving in another shantytown somewhere in Zimbabwe. *Two steps backward rather than one step forward. We did what we thought was best, but it wasn't enough.*

*

Our 3½-month "trial" to see if we wanted to again do long-term missionary work was soon at an end. A resounding "yes" was the answer. Just like at Silveira, I was soon deeply involved in all aspects of the hospital, and even though the AIDS problem was daunting, maybe there was a glimmer of hope. We had started a "mother to child prevention" program and were having some success. It was a small but important *"step along the way,"* and that step would eventually lead us to a successful AIDS treatment program. We left Zimbabwe in January 2002 to attend the wedding of our youngest son

Tim, returning in April for another seven years. *I really enjoy the work at the hospital, and we fit into the Mission Complex quite well. Still, it's hard trying to understand the culture better. I'm so impatient and get upset way too often. The laissez-faire attitude of some of the hospital staff "runs me up the wall"—especially when it comes to distributing patient meds. When mistakes are made, it seems it's always someone else's fault. Still, all in all, the staff are hard working and want to do the best for the patients. I need patience, patience, patience.*

AIDS

May 2002:

I walked into the overcrowded Women's Ward to make rounds on 48 patients. As I entered the first ward, ten beds were shoved together where six should fit, the smell of sickness was overwhelming, a smell that doctors know so well. A smell that screams that death is around the corner, and for some, the corner is only a few feet away. In some wards, sickness permeated the room like a steamroller overwhelming all in its path, and in others the smell was hidden by strong disinfectant odors, but the underlying stench of death came wafting through to my sensitive nose.

All the normal beds were occupied, plus seven overflow beds in the hallway. Most patients had various opportunistic infections related to AIDS. I was a bit out of sorts because I was the only doctor at this 165-bed hospital. Before we left St. Theresa's for the U.S. in Mid-January, I heard a rumor that Dr. Tsododo—my Zimbabwean colleague—might be moving to Driefontein Mission to receive surgical training from Dr. Aschwanden. To see if it was true, I directly asked him, "Dr. Tsododo, are you going to be here when I return in April?"

"Yes, I'll be here."

I think he feared I might not return *if* I was going to be alone at this busy hospital—and he may have been right. Maybe he thought this "little white lie" was warranted under the circumstances. He wanted me to return, and knew that once here, I would stay even if alone.

He didn't stay and I was alone—and overwhelmed by the sheer number of sick and dying patients. I stood there looking at the crowded Women's Ward: *"Am I really up to this? Do I really want to be this busy? Can I handle this at age 65? I know I had the energy and enthusiasm in my 30's, but in my 60's? What have I gotten myself into? Well, Doctor, get to work. It's not going to get done by itself."*

I was facing a large number of AIDS patients with very little experience in treating them, and to make matters worse, I didn't have any anti-viral medicines. All I could do was treat the various opportunistic infections associated with AIDS and hope to add a few months to their lives.

Victoria was in the first bed, 33 years old, little more than a skeleton. Not a walking skeleton because she was totally bed-ridden. AIDS is called "slimming disease" by the Africans, and people with advanced AIDS certainly are slim—not just slim, but cadaverous. She was five-feet tall and weighed 65 pounds. She looked at me with a "deer in the headlights" look that I had seen so often since my arrival—a wide-eyed, frightened, and anxious look that said to me "I'm scared. Is there any hope?" Sadly, there wasn't. The only thing I could do was treat whatever infection she might have and hope she would get better for a short time. Otherwise, our only treatment was to provide hospice care for the dying.

Standing next to Victoria was her 13-year-old daughter. She was helping her mother and hoping we were going to do something to cure her. Her father died the previous year from AIDS, and a four-year-old brother died six months later. There were three other siblings at home. This girl looked healthy. I figured she probably was born before her father brought the virus home and shared it with her mother, who then passed it on to the lastborn child. We didn't have tests available to diagnose AIDS so we did it the old fashioned way, on a clinical basis. In most cases there was no doubt. When Victoria would die—not IF, because she was certainly going to die soon—this 13-year-old girl would likely be the primary caregiver for her siblings. She would have to do the cooking and washing and bathing and farming, hoping to get a bit of assistance from the neighbors and maybe from the good Sisters at St. Theresa's. She certainly wouldn't be able to go to school. Too young to have so much responsibility, but we saw similar social situations every day. Our Home Based Care program assisted AIDS patients who were dying at home, and then gave as much help as possible to the orphans who were left behind. With no effective treatment options, the number of orphans throughout the District was increasing faster than our Home Based Care program could possibly absorb. *What to do? What to do?* The "Romero Prayer" says, "You can't do everything, but *you can do something and do it very well." But right now, there doesn't seem to be anything to do except help people die. Is that all I can do? Come on God, you've got to show me the way. There has to be a way to start an AIDS treatment program.*

Victoria was ill this time with diarrhea. She had been hospitalized three times in the past four months, and each admission recorded a lower weight. Her immune system was almost non-existent, and soon she would get a fatal infection. I was trying to adjust her medicines to help the diarrhea so she could go home for a few more months—or maybe not. After listening to her lungs and examining her abdomen, I gave a small, thin-lipped smile to the daughter and moved on.

Beatrice was in the next bed, with a high fever and cough. Her x-ray showed severe pneumonia, hopefully one that would respond to high doses of penicillin. She was only 22, also gaunt, also that now familiar "deer in the headlights" look. She worked in Harare as a secretary. Her married boyfriend who gave her the virus, died last year. Fortunately, she didn't have any children. Her mother gave me that same worried look and asked, "Can't you please do something for Beatrice?"

I sadly shook my head, "I'm doing all I can. Maybe the penicillin will help."

The next bed had screens around it, with a flurry of activity going on behind the screens. I peered in and the nurse said, "She just died. We're getting ready to move her to the mortuary." We were averaging one or two deaths per day. Our six-bed mortuary frequently had 12 or more bodies, waiting for relatives to come and take them home for burial. Coffin-making businesses in the nearby township—and throughout the country—were some of the busiest enterprises in a country of massive unemployment.

The nurse asked, "Could you please complete the death certificate now? The brother wants to go to the authorities for a burial order." In filling out the form, I could not put "AIDS" as the cause of death. It wasn't politically correct. Not acceptable. People were still refusing to believe that such a disease existed. It was like leprosy in Biblical times. They would talk about "slim disease" or "that illness" or "you know, the usual thing," but never mention AIDS. I wrote "I.S.D." as the cause of death—meaning "Immune System Disease." That actually is an accurate description of the cause of death, because AIDS destroys the immune system so people die from T.B., or meningitis, or pneumonia, or sarcoma, or diarrhea, but not *directly* from the AIDS virus.

Before I left the ward, a nurse and five student nurses started to wheel the shrouded body out of the ward. As they entered the hallway, relatives started to moan and weep, a few of them loudly keening, and the sad entourage slowly made its way to the mortuary, the student nurses staring straight ahead with tear-filled eyes. And so it went, day after day, the same heavy-hearted procession; on some days, several processions. Just as in the 70's when there were frequent deaths from measles and whooping cough, I became hardened to the frequent AIDS deaths. Many of the patients died before I even saw them, or had only been in the hospital a few days so I really didn't get to know them. I tried my best to get them over one more infection, but to no avail. I couldn't let myself become emotionally involved—it was just too painful. And yet, the nurses and students were emotionally involved and crying with each death. Some days it seemed too much to bear.

Monica was next. Fortunately, not *all* patients had AIDS. She looked healthy and came in with a high fever, most likely due to malaria. She had recently been to visit relatives in the Lowveld area where malaria was endemic. The admitting nurse started her on appropriate malaria treatment. Her temperature was normal and she had a pretty smile on her face. "How are you today, Monica?"

"Fine doctor."

"Do you want to go home?"

Bigger smile, "Yes."

"Fine. The nurse will give you some medicine to take at home."

With a smile on my face, I wrote the discharge orders. I felt good to know that there were still a few patients we could "cure" and send home healthy. I was tired of being depressed about so many AIDS patients dying. So many very ill patients and so little I could do. It reminded me of the measles and whooping cough patients in the 70's, but this was worse. Instead of 30 to 40 people dying per year, we were having that number every month. I was hoping that maybe we could do something as exciting for AIDS patients as we did back then. No vaccines were available, but maybe, just maybe, we would find some treatment options.

Anna, age 28, weighed 70 pounds. Her x-ray showed extensive T.B. She had been on treatment for three weeks, and was slowly improving. She looked better but not ready for discharge. T.B. had been coming under control in Zimbabwe until the onset of the AIDS epidemic. Since 1990, the rate skyrocketed. Many with quiescent T.B. activated their disease as their immune system faltered. The only good news was that we had excellent medicines for T.B. and many dramatically improved on treatment, only to later succumb to other opportunistic infections. AIDS is relentless—it always wins if there is not effective treatment against the virus, and at that time, I had no treatment. Still, Anna was getting better, was slowly gaining weight, and with a gap-toothed smile on her face, she asked, "When can I go home, doctor?"

"Another two or three weeks, Anna."

"Thank you."

Charity was 26. At one time she was probably a beautiful woman, but now it was difficult to look at a face that was grotesquely disfigured by an ugly black fungating tumor near her left eye. The eye was swollen closed. Kaposi Sarcoma was an uncommon cancer before the AIDS epidemic, but now it was common, and we had no treatment. It seemed as if you could watch it grow, as it changed from day to day. It was not only on her face, but also in her lungs, and most likely spread throughout her body. The only thing I had for Charity was a bit of oral morphine for pain and the prayers of the Sister chaplain.

I trudged through the Women's Ward until it was time for tea, one of the traditions that remained since our time in the 70's. Ten A.M. was teatime, and everyone—and I mean everyone— stopped for a break. The only exception was if I was in the midst of an operation. In that case, I would finish the surgery and *then* have tea. I walked down the slight hill to our house to have tea and biscuits (cookies) with Loretta. I needed the respite. We could talk about other things to get my mind away from the huge number of ill and dying AIDS patients. *Try to get back to "normal," even in the midst of disaster. Personal war stories have revealed how soldiers would talk about the most inane things in the midst of battle while crouching low in a foxhole or trench. I could not continuously focus on AIDS. I needed to have other outlets or I would go mad worrying about why I wasn't doing something to help the situation.*

On to the Male Ward—same thing; then to the Children's Ward—same thing. In fact, the children's ward was even more depressing. Seeing one-year-olds and two-year-olds and five-year-olds dying of AIDS—*dear God, what am I to do?*

Talent was one of the five-year-olds. He had T.B. of his lungs and fluid around his heart, all due to AIDS. He weighed just 20 pounds and could barely stand. Still, he looked at me with a big smile on his face. *How can you smile at me when you're so sick?*

"Talent, how are you today?"

Proudly showing off his English and emphasizing each and every word, he replied, "I – am – fine – dock-o-tor. How – are - you?"

"I am fine. Let me listen to your heart." I had drained half a pint of fluid from around his heart the day before, and he was some better. He wasn't coughing as much and his breathing was easier. Maybe he would get better with the T.B. drugs? Even if I got him over the T.B., I still worried that Talent would die before we had drugs available to treat his AIDS virus. Usually people improved on T.B. treatment, and might even get well enough to live another two or three years with AIDS—maybe long enough for us to start a treatment program at St. Theresa's? I hoped so.

The only relief from the onslaught of AIDS patients was the O.B. ward. It was still populated with mostly non-HIV patients. With a sigh of relief I walked onto the ward to see the smiling face of a mother with a newborn baby at her breast. In the hallway were ten women with blue hospital gowns, sitting with their babies—each baby wearing a knitted cap and colorful baby clothes—listening to a talk on the proper feeding of their infants. They all greeted me, "Masikati Dockotor." (Good afternoon Doctor).

"Masikati, madzimai. Makidii? (Good afternoon, mothers. How are you?)"

"Tiripo (We are fine.)"

"Munofara here? (Are you happy?)"

"Tinofara chaiizvo (We are very happy.)"

Indeed, the maternity ward was one of the happiest places in the hospital. When I needed a bit of cheering up, I would drop in there, sit for a while to chat with a nurse, and watch the joyful mothers with their newborn babies. The nurses were in a better mood because they didn't have to care for sick and dying patients. Every six months we had a rotation of where the nurses worked, and those moving to maternity were the most happy to be moved. Three or four times a month I was called to do a Caesarian Section—another delightful event since it nearly always resulted in a healthy crying baby and a smiling mother.

It's not to say that there wasn't HIV on the OB department. When we arrived in 2001, the incidence of HIV in pregnant mothers was 25 to 30%, but most of them were in the early stages of AIDS. They weren't showing the normal illnesses of AIDS, but they still could transmit the virus to their unborn baby, and even if it was negative at birth, they likely would transmit it in breast milk, and that was the only option for poor rural women.

After lunch, it was time to face the horde of outpatients. As I walked to my office, there were at least 35 people sitting on the benches. It would be a long afternoon. Florence, a surgical assistant who also worked in outpatient, was my interpreter that day. I was glad to have her because she didn't try to "interpret" in a manner to please me, but just gave me what the patient actually said. She was usually in a good mood and I liked to tease her. We got along well.

"Good afternoon, Florence. How's your love life?"

Shyly, "Good afternoon doctor. Not so good. My boyfriend just left for South Africa to find work, and I don't know if I'll see him again."

"Sorry to hear that. Guess I'm going to have to find someone for you—someone rich, who can take you away from all of this, right?"

Giggling, she answered, "Oh, please do."

"Well, I'll look around for you. Right now we better start working to get through this long line of patients."

Peter was first. He was in a wheelchair, unable to stand or walk. Once again, those familiar "deer in the headlights" look. Thin. Confused. Coughing. Horrific rash. No confusion about the diagnosis—far-advanced AIDS. I quickly examined him, wrote orders to admit, got an x-ray and blood count, and started antibiotics. Not much hope, at least not any long-term hope. Maybe he had something that would respond to antibiotics, and he might have a few more months, but not more than that.

Julia, age 70, was next. Not AIDS, but still not good. She was in a wheelchair because of a recent stroke. She was unable to speak, unable to stand, had paralysis of her right hand and leg, and was incontinent of urine—a difficult management problem in the U.S., but nearly impossible in rural Africa. The family had been caring for her at home, changing underclothes and cleaning her, trying to get her to take a bit of food and drink, turning her in bed. They finally brought her to the hospital because she had a large pressure sore on her left buttock. Again I reached for the admission sheet. We could not keep patients for long-term care, but I would try to get the sore to heal, and then instruct the family in better care at home.

And so it went. Day after day of making rounds on dying AIDS patients, then seeing more of them in outpatient. No good treatment. Watching them die. Frustrated and depressed. What to do? Is that all we could do?—be a "step along the way" to help so many people die? The U.N. had a new program to help poor countries develop treatment programs. The new UNAIDS slogan of "Five by 2005" described their goal of five million people on AIDS treatment by 2005. Maybe we could get some of that help?

*

In early 2001, a serendipitous meeting led to the first step of developing a "Mother-to-Child Prevention" program at St. Theresa's. Sister Patricia, that same Irish Dominican Nun fireball who met us at the airport in October '01, and who helped me find Loretta when she was "lost," and who visited us at Silveira in the 70's to study our approach to community medicine and the prevention of measles and whooping cough and malnutrition, and who took our program and greatly expanded it over the next ten years at St. Theresa Hospital, was at a meeting with Dr. Peter Iliff discussing HIV in the Harare area. Peter was a pediatrician who worked with ZVITAMBO (acronym for "Zimbabwe Vitamin A for Mothers and Babies Project"), a Non-Governmental-Organization that had just completed a large research project in Harare on the transmission of HIV from mother to child.

Peter lamented to Sister Pat, "We're having trouble finding a rural hospital partner. We want to continue our work in prevention of mother-to-child transmission in a rural area, but so far haven't found one willing to take on the responsibility and work with us."

"I know just the place," Sr. Pat told him. Because she was on the Board of Directors for St. Theresa Hospital, she could make things happen, and she did. Within a few weeks, meetings were arranged and a partnership was forged—a partnership that continued for 15 years.

With their help, we finally were able to test pregnant women for HIV. ZVITAMBO also provided medication to give newborn babies born of HIV positive mothers, medicine that helped to prevent the babies from getting the virus. A small "first step."

As with any new program, it required cajoling and training of the O.B. staff, most of whom were resistant to change. "We're already too busy." "We don't have the time." "We should get paid more if we have to do more." "It won't make any difference, anyway." Still, they were keen to have additional training to get one more certificate to hang on the wall, so we progressed with training and then to implementation—testing all pregnant mothers who agreed to be tested, and giving them "pre-test" and "post-test counseling."

Even though this was a "baby step," it became a huge step. Within a year we were rolling out the program, and within two years, we were able to test whoever agreed to be tested. The biggest change was that we finally were getting people to accept they had the AIDS virus and should do something about it: safe sex; have their other children tested; talk about being HIV positive; live positively with HIV; *have their husband tested;* attend antenatal clinic regularly; deliver at the hospital so the baby could be treated soon after delivery. Within a year of implementation, the "Mother-to-Child" prevention was merely another part of normal O.B. care, just like taking blood pressure, weighing the mother, or palpating the abdomen to determine the position of the baby. It has always amazed me that we can be so resistant to change, but when we start doing it and seeing the results, it becomes such an easy part of routine care.

The next step was to develop a treatment program for our staff members who were sick with AIDS. With a staff of 90 and a national incidence of 25%, at least 20 of our staff most likely had HIV, and 5 or 10 might be ill with AIDS. Two of them had recently died at home without being tested. IF some of the of the staff were willing to come forward, we would use donor funds to privately purchase anti-retroviral drugs at a cost of U.S. $30 per month, and start them on treatment. In April 2004, Finance Mutero became one of the first. At five feet ten, she was a large vivacious woman who worked in our Home-Based-Care (HBC) department, helping coordinate home-care for those dying of AIDS. She was tested for HIV during her last pregnancy and found to be positive. Her newborn daughter was treated soon after birth, and remained HIV negative. Now, Finance was separated from her alcoholic, abusive, philandering husband and had the responsibility for her three children. I saw her in my office for a second visit to talk about AIDS treatment.

"Do you want to start AIDS treatment?" She was in Clinical Stage III (of four clinical stages, with Four being the sickest) and would be a good candidate for treatment.

"Yes. I'm losing a lot of weight. I keep getting colds and I don't have much energy. My kids need me because their father's no good and won't look after them if I die."

"Last time we talked about the risks of the medicines. Do you understand those risks?"

"Yes. I know there's risk, but I still want to take it. It's my only hope."

"OK. Here's what we'll do. I'll give you this one-month supply of 'three drugs in one pill.' You take one in the morning and one in the evening every day, never missing. It's extremely important to not miss any doses. Let me know immediately if you have any side effect. Do you understand?"

"Yes."

Finance became a spokeswoman for "people living with AIDS (PLWA's)." She openly talked about her disease and treatment at large group meetings. She was well known throughout the District, and people could see how she went from being very ill to being completely healthy. She gained 50 pounds, so at one follow-up visit, I said, "Finance, you have to start watching your diet. You're gaining too much weight!"

With a nervous laugh, she said, "I know doctor, but I just feel so good and everything tastes so good. I feel totally alive once again. I'm so happy, I just can't help but eat when food is available."

Her bravery of facing the community stigma by speaking about AIDS went a long way to break down barriers so others would eventually step forward for treatment and speak out in the same brave manner. We later tested her second youngest, four-year-old Vimbai, and found her to be positive and in need of treatment. Today, they are both healthy—seventeen years after starting treatment

With that "second step" in our AIDS treatment program, and since Finance stepped forward so publicly, we had several staff members come to me for treatment. Then, a few private patients who could afford the $30 per month started asking for "that medicine." One of them was Monica, 30 years old, admitted with pneumonia and weighing only 60 pounds. Two family members accompanied her. When her pneumonia started to improve, they came to me and asked, "Can't you start her on AIDS treatment?"

I knew she came from far away, so I told them, "You come from too far. How can I be sure she will come back every month for follow-up?"

"We'll make certain she returns. We promise. Please help her."

"Can you afford to pay the $30 each and every month?"

"Several of her relatives have jobs and will help pay. We have $60 now for two months, and can have that amount every two months."

"That's easy to say today because you have the money. What happens if you can't get it?"

"Doctor, we'll get it. If necessary, we'll sell a cow or two. We have a herd of 30 at home, so there won't be any problem."

"Monica, do you want treatment?"

"Yes."

"You know, you're still very ill and might die before the medicine starts to work. It takes three to six months to be effective. Maybe we're starting too late." From experience, I knew that in very ill patients, up to 50% would die during the first few months. Still, 50% were surviving. Without treatment, over 95% would be dead in one year and 100% in two years. If we were treating a Stage 4 cancer that had a 95% one-year mortality, and now had a treatment with 50% recovery rate, everyone would think we had a miracle drug. To me, that's what anti-retroviral treatment was—a miracle.

"Yes, I know the risks. I want to take the pills. Otherwise I die for sure."

We started Monica on treatment in the hospital. She gradually improved, going home six weeks later weighing 65 pounds. Because she lived far from the hospital, I had reservations about treating her, but due to family pressure, I acquiesced and glad that I did. She became a "poster woman" for AIDS treatment, returning every month and then every two months, never missing an appointment. A year later I was walking by the AIDS follow-up clinic, and a woman shouted, "Doctor, don't you recognize me?"

"No, I don't. Who are you?"

"Monica, from Chiredzi."

"Monica. I can't believe it. You look wonderful. How are you feeling?"

"I'm so good and so happy. Look at me." With white teeth gleaming in a big smile shining on her happy face, she turned around and around to show me that she was the picture of health. She had gained 60 pounds. Imagine, in one year, she had doubled her weight. With that huge smile she was openly telling everyone she had recovered from AIDS. If she had been a male, I would have nicknamed her "Lazarus" because she truly had risen from the dead. Elise Frederick, CEO of our Mission Doctors Association, later said to me, "Can you imagine ANY woman being happy about gaining 60 pounds?" I could imagine it because I saw it time after time.

George was another poster man for treatment success. He had been working in Botswana, knew he had AIDS, but couldn't afford the treatment. He came to us with severe headache and barely able to talk. Spinal fluid showed he had Cryptococcal meningitis, a normally uncommon fungal infection of the brain but fairly common in Stage Four AIDS patients. The anti-fungal treatment is very expensive (over $300 U.S. per month), but Pfizer Pharmaceutical arranged to make it free for many countries in Africa. We were lucky enough to have a supply. I started George on Diflucan treatment, and he rapidly improved.

"George, you're much better. Now you need AIDS treatment. What should we do? I can't treat you if you work in Botswana."

"Doctor, I want to be treated. Even though I work in Botswana, I really live in Gweru (a two hour bus trip away), and I'll return every month if necessary."

"George, aren't you going back to Botswana?"

"It's a good job, but my health comes first. I'll stay in Gweru and come here every month."

Before he left the hospital, we tested George's wife. She was HIV negative. That was good news. Although not common, it also was not rare that a spouse of a patient with full-blown AIDS would be HIV negative—so far, they had just been lucky. It reinforced the need for condom use whenever they had sex, so the virus would not be spread to his wife. I didn't look on condom use as a "pregnancy prevention method," but rather as a "life saving method."

George returned monthly for several months. One day I saw him in the follow-up clinic. "You look good, George. How're you feeling?"

"Great doctor. But, I have to return to work in Botswana to support my family. There's no work in Zimbabwe, and I can make good money as a mechanic in Francistown, just across the border."

"What are you going to do about your medicines?"

"If you give me a two month supply, then I'll be sure to come home every two months and come here. I promise." And he did. For the next seven years he came every two months, and reliably took his medicines, and continued to do well. Even though I was skeptical, he proved me wrong and proved that we could treat *some* patients even though they came from far away.

Eric was another miracle. He came to the hospital paralyzed below the waist, cadaverous, and one more patient with that "deer in the headlights" look. He had far-advanced Stage IV AIDS, and I doubted that any treatment was going to help him, but because his family insisted, we started him on treatment. Although he slowly gained some weight, there was no improvement in his legs. Each week as I saw him, I would ask, "Eric, how are you today?"

"Getting better, doctor."

"Can you move your toes?" He would grimace and try everything to move them, but nothing happened. Month after month, no improvement, and then one day there was slight movement in his big toe. Over several weeks, there was movement in the other foot and then in both legs. Our physical therapist worked with him. Eventually he was able to stand and then slowly to walk, using a walker.

"Eric, you look great. Do you want to go home?"

"Oh, yes doctor."

"Who's going to help you at home?" I knew his wife had left him and returned to her family home some distance away, and she wasn't coming back. His two sons lived with him, one 14 and one 6.

Patrick, the fourteen year old was there, and answered, "I'll be there and I'll look after him."

"Don't you go to school?"

"No. It's more important I take care of him."

"What do you think, Eric?"

"He's a good boy. He'll take care of me."

Sister Andrea visited Eric several times at his home since he had no way to come to the hospital. She refilled his meds, made sure he didn't have any bedsores or other problems, and gave me reports on how well he was doing. I decided to go with her one day to see for myself.

Driving over one of the worst roads in the District, we bumped and jerked over huge holes, drove over a few under water bridges, up steep sandy embankments, and finally we were close enough to walk a half-mile to Eric's home. Greeting him as we approached, "Eric, we are approaching."

"Please enter," said Eric.

He was inside a round, thatched-roof hut. Only a bit of daylight filtered in, so our eyes had to adjust to the darkness of the hut. He was lying on a low bed with Patrick beside him.

After the normal greetings, I asked, "Are you really getting better?"

"Oh yes, doctor. Each week I get a bit stronger. Now I can get up by myself and walk to the toilet, and sit outside. Patrick has made a garden. He does all my work. I hope that with time, I'll be able to do it."

With that, Eric slowly got out of bed, grabbed the walker, and walked outside to sit on a stump in front of his hut. He had nothing, and yet he had everything. No water, no electricity, no refrigeration, only a pit toilet. And yet, he was happy—as happy as if he had just won the lottery and was the richest man in the District. Of course, he had won the lottery of AIDS treatment, and now had won his health back. Hopefully, with more time, he would walk normally and be able to do his own farming and gardening.

"Patrick, you've done an excellent job taking care of your father. I'm sure he's proud of you. I know I am."

"Thanks doctor."

"Where is Joyful, your young brother?"

"He's at school, but should be back soon."

"We have to get back to the hospital, so be sure to greet him for us. Goodbye Eric and Patrick."

"Goodbye doctor and Sister."

Just as I started the car, Joyful came bounding up the road with a huge grin. "Doctor, doctor. Sister, Sister, wait." He jumped into Sister's lap and started jabbering in Shona, the joy of his name written all over his face.

*

In such a manner, we developed a small but effective treatment program. When the Ministry of Health came to see if we were ready to receive UNAIDS Global Fund drugs, we had everything in order and were quickly approved. Soon we were starting 30 to 40 AIDS patients on treatment each month. From the "one small step" of preventing transmission from mother to baby, we took several small steps until we had a full-fledged treatment program, and became an example for other rural mission hospitals to follow.

Just as in the 1970's, we found that if we wanted to provide treatment to all the AIDS patients in our District, we would have to develop out-stations for treatment. Eventually we developed four sites that we visited each month. New patients were tested and if they met our criteria, were started on treatment at those centers.

By July 2014, St. Theresa Hospital had started more than 3,300 patients on treatment. Many have died because of starting too late in their disease process. Some have defaulted treatment, but not nearly as many as we expected. I believe that compliance is better in rural Africa than in much of the "developed world"—there are *fewer* distractions! Some 2,500 remain on treatment and are totally well.

Experts in AIDS treatment tell us that *if* a person is compliant with their treatment and don't miss doses, they can live long and productive lives. Their immune systems return to normal, and they die of "natural causes" rather than from opportunistic infections.

In the St. Theresa Hospital District there has been a dramatic decrease in the incidence of new AIDS cases, a decrease in the infectivity of those on treatment, and most importantly, a dramatic decrease in AIDS related deaths. There are fewer new cases of T.B., meningitis, pneumonia, diarrhea, Kaposi Sarcoma, and other opportunistic infections.

The hospital census decreased from an average of 120 patients per day in 2001 to 60 patients per day in 2009. The overall incidence of AIDS in the country went from 25% in 2002 to 14% in 2009—still far too high, but trending in the right direction. The incidence of transmission from mother to child at St. Theresa Hospital went from 50% in 2000 to 10% in 2011.

There's still more to do, but that "first step" many years ago led to many more steps along the way to helping those with full-blown AIDS. This came about because the entire staff slowly but surely bought into the aspect that prevention of spread from mother to child was important, and then believed that if everyone worked together, we could develop a successful AIDS treatment program. It was not easy. There were many stumbling blocks along the way, but with perseverance, we slowly developed a successful program. To me, there was nothing more satisfying than to work in the follow-up clinic and see the many people who came for refills. To see that big smile and receive a huge "thank you" from patient after patient who had been near death, but now had gained 30 or 40 or even 60 pounds, and were completely well. Instead of feeling frustrated and depressed, I was elated and energized. Maybe I should be called Lazarus, because my spirits and enthusiasm had been re-born.

By email in April 2013, I received information about Finance Mutero, that first staff member we started on AIDS treatment. Besides giving permission to use her story in this book, she sent the following:

"Nowadays I am doing well, only that I am not getting any salary and there is hunger. This is really a problem to both of us because the medication increases appetite and we have nothing to eat and it causes discomfort to take tablets on an empty stomach. I feel sorry for my child who goes to school without enough food. I am not managing to pay fees for my children as well as buying food for them.

"My weight was 120 pounds when I started treatment and now I am 170. I started treatment on 12 May 2004 and my daughter on 14 June 2005. When I started treatment I only had one side effect—one of swelling of face. Up to now I don't have any problems with medication.

"My CD4 (a blood count that measures immune cells) was 37 when I started treatment and now its 702 and Vimbai my daughter had a CD4 count of 199 when she started; now its 750. She is now in Form 3 and she is always taking her drugs. She is actually the one who reminds me to take my drugs. She looks very fit. We usually talk about HIV/AIDS both of us as well as with the other children. The last born who comes after Vimbai is negative. I joined PMTCT when I realized that I was pregnant with the last one. I spend most of my time doing counseling to my daughter Vimbai because I feel that she constantly needs it.

"I have also realized and I do believe that drug adherence is very important and I also feel that I am benefiting from the AIDS treatment I wouldn't be alive otherwise."

HELP IS ON THE WAY

From April 2002 to January 2003, I was the only doctor at St. Theresa's. With each passing month, I could feel my energy and enthusiasm leaking away like water seeping from a bucket with a hole in the bottom. In November, after another long day of making rounds on a third of the 140 patients, doing two emergency C-sections, and then facing the seemingly endless line of outpatients, I slowly trudged my way home. Grabbing a Lion Lager from the fridge, I joined Loretta on the verandah, took a large satisfying gulp of beer and exhaled a long slow "Aaaah."

Loretta looked up and said, "That bad, huh?"

"Yep, another day and another dollar and no help on the horizon. Wow, I'm tired. I blew up at one of the nurses in outpatients this afternoon for no reason at all. I'm becoming more short-tempered and crankier, and I don't want to be remembered as 'the angry old man.' I hope the Sisters find help soon."

The hospital work was never completely done, but when the end of the workday came, whatever was left had to wait until tomorrow. My title was "Medical Superintendent." Although it sounds impressive, what it really meant was more work, especially in the administration area. When I was in my 30's I thrived on such a schedule, but at 65 it was too much—too many patients to see, too many "administration" hassles, too many interruptions, too many months of being on call "24-7." This was retirement? On our arrival in April we told the Dominican Sisters we would stay "as long as our health and energy lasted." As the year dragged on, it became apparent neither would last *if* relief wasn't found, and found soon.

"The latest rumor is that Sister / Doctor Clara Jeketera *might* be coming in January. I don't know what I'll do if she doesn't." Doctor Clara was a Dominican Nun who "grew into the medical profession" after joining the Dominican Order when she was eighteen. After two years as a "Candidate" and three more as a "Novice," she worked within the Dominican organization as a newly professed Sister. After finishing a pre-Medical course, she attended medical school at the University of Zimbabwe, did the standard two-year internship, and most recently had spent two years being the only doctor at Regina Coeli Hospital near the Mozambique border.

When I first met Clara at a Hospital Board meeting in January 2002, she gave me the ultimate compliment. After greeting each other, she said, "I've frequently heard Sister Patricia tell how you instigated the measles vaccination program in the Bikita District in the 1970's. I might be alive today because of your work, because I grew up in the town of Bikita, and when I was four my mother took me to be immunized at one of your clinics."

Twenty-seven years after leaving Rhodesia I was getting positive feedback. Part of the "Romero Prayer" says " . . . We may never see the end result, but that is the difference between the master builder and the worker . . . ," but this time I did see an end result and it was rewarding. This talented African woman, Nun, doctor, and soon-to-be-friend was standing in front of me as proof positive that measles vaccination saved lives. Her complement was one of those "warm fuzzies" we all cherish when they come our way.

Sister / Doctor Clara did arrive in early January. Whew! What a relief to have someone sharing the workload, to be there to discuss diagnoses and treatments and to help with surgery. As you might imagine, with so many sick patients in the hospital, we were both busy, and when one was on vacation or at a seminar, the other was once again alone. Doctor Clara was near the age I was when at Silveira and she had that same energy and enthusiasm. Shortly after her arrival she encouraged me to take some long weekends away from the hospital, so in late January, Loretta and I had a four-day weekend at Norma Jean's Lake View Resort overlooking Lake Mtirikwi (known to us as Lake Kyle in the 1970's.)

Norma Jean's was an all-inclusive resort, so it meant four days of sleeping late, lounging, reading, resting, listening to a multitude of birds in the beautifully managed flower gardens, watching the sunset over Lake Mtirikwi with a sun-downer of gin and tonic in hand, eating too much, and recuperating. No cooking for Loretta, no patients for me to see, no people coming to our gate to ask for help, no telephone calls. Once again, *I felt human! And best of all, I was on call only every other week.*

With two of us sharing the load, 2003 went smoothly and my crankiness subsided a notch. In January 2004, Dr. Tim Cavanaugh, recently retired from the U.S. Indian Health Service, and his wife, Sheila, arrived from Los Angeles. Like us, they were recruited, trained, and supported by Mission Doctors Association. It was a Godsend to have another Yankee couple on the mission. Although we were the only Yanks for the 4½ years we spent at Silveira in the 1970's, it didn't feel like being alone because we were kept busy with our seven children. Now we felt a certain loneliness, even though Dr. Clara had been working with me for the past year. She was a great help at the hospital and we got along well, but she was part of the Dominican community. Though we were always welcomed by everyone on the mission and never felt excluded, we still felt the social and cultural differences.

Why is that? We got along well with everyone and easily made friends. Loretta started a "prayer group" of local women who met weekly to pray for school children, and she became close friends with many of those women. We socialized with the Dominican Sisters and the religious staff at the Mission, but never really felt part of them—not because of them, but because of us, or more accurately, because of me. When we had some of the Zimbabwe staff to our house for dinner or a social evening, it felt a bit awkward and forced. There wasn't that easy camaraderie we felt when playing bridge with a group of friends in Wisconsin. Never the same back and forth bantering and kidding. Different cultures and different social customs? I sometimes felt that people came to our events "because I was the boss at the hospital" and not because they really wanted to come. At the hospital, the social interactions between the staff and me were easy and seldom strained—except when I was yelling or screaming because medicines weren't given or patients didn't receive proper care. The easy interaction was especially true when the entire surgical crew sat around for tea and bread and jam after a difficult case. The ebb and flow of talk and gossip was similar to when I worked at the Shawano Hospital in Wisconsin. Maybe the common hospital work made us all more "equal," but when people visited us or we visited them, they didn't feel "equal?" I don't know, but wish it had been easier for us. With Tim and Sheila, we immediately established an easy rapport and quickly became close friends. If we only could have had that same type of relationship with Dr. George in 1970, our time at Driefontein would have been so much more enjoyable.

We met Tim and Sheila at the airport as they arrived in Harare. Tim was going to have to work for two months at a hospital in Harare to learn how to do C-sections—something he easily could have learned in two weeks, but the government hospital cherished the "free help." We were there to welcome them to Zimbabwe and be sure they felt appreciated and needed, and let them know we would be available if there were any problems during their time in Harare.

"Welcome to Zimbabwe," Loretta and I shouted as they came through the customs area.

"Thank you," they both replied as we shook hands and hugged. Tim said, "We've heard a lot about you during our classes in Los Angeles."

"All of it bad, I'm sure."

"No, all of it good. You have a lot to live up to."

"I'm afraid you'll quickly see all our warts and blemishes. It's hard to hide anything on the Mission."

"We'll see."

After loading their luggage into the back of our Isuzu Double Cab Pickup, we drove from the airport towards the center of Harare. It was a beautiful summer day, temperature in the 80's, little humidity, and clear skies. The skyscrapers in the distance looked like a modern Capitol City, but the trash along the road, the beggars on every street corner, the many deep potholes, and the inoperative traffic lights belied that impression. I said, "Yes, the city is dirty. There's not enough money for garbage collection or street repairs. You'll be glad to leave Harare and come out into the bush with us when you finish at the hospital."

"What about Harare Hospital?" asked Tim.

"They're struggling. It's the same problem of not enough money to buy supplies."

"And St. Theresa's?"

"Because of generous donors, we are much better than any of the government hospitals. Still, we struggle, but we do have the basic supplies we need."

Later that evening, as we sat around relaxing, I said to Tim, "I've read your C.V., and see you were born in Maquoketa, Iowa?"

"Yes. We lived in DeWitt, but Maquoketa was the nearest hospital."

"I was born there too."

"No way! In Maquoketa?"

"Yes, but when I was two, we moved to Farley."

Sheila said, "Farley? I grew up in Dubuque, and I have a cousin living in Farley." It's only 20 miles West of Dubuque, and during my teenage years I made many trips to dances at Melody Mill in Dubuque. One frequently hears "It's a small world," but who would imagine that two U. S. mission doctors would meet for the first time in Zimbabwe and find they were born in the same small town in Iowa?

After Tim spent his obligatory two months working at the huge Charity Hospital in Harare, they moved to St. Theresa's and were with us for the next three years. I saw Tim every day at the hospital and he was of immeasurable help in all aspects of medicine. On many days I would look for him, and say, "Tim, come and look at this patient and let me know what you think about her x-ray." After perusing the x-ray and then examining the patient, he would offer his advice and we would discuss treatment options. He was one of the most knowledgeable Family Practice doctors I've ever known. If he didn't know the answer, he had a program on his computer that would find it for us. Besides being a good doctor, he was also a computer geek. He knew *everything* about computers, so whenever one of the hospital computers was causing problems, I would tell Ms Hove, "Find Doctor Cavanaugh. He'll fix it for you," and he would.

He was a hard worker at the hospital—sometimes I thought he worked too hard. One day I took him aside and said, "Tim, I know you think you need to spend all that time at the hospital, but the nurses don't want you around after 5:00 PM, and Sheila needs you at home. Why don't you try that?" I knew that each of us could spend 24 hours a day at the hospital and still not get all the work done, so it was necessary to compartmentalize and do what we could during a normal work day. The patients would still be there tomorrow.

Being Tim, he easily agreed. That's the way he was—easy going, willing to help with anything, hard working, and smart. Loretta enjoyed having Sheila nearby as a friend and confidant. They frequently had morning coffee together to catch up on hospital and mission gossip, went shopping, helped each other with projects, and Sheila joined Loretta's weekly prayer group.

Shortly after they arrived, Loretta and Sheila drove to Masvingo on a shopping trip. It was Sheila's first foray into the world of small-town

Zimbabwe shopping. Loretta was comfortable driving our Isuzu Pickup, so the two of them were off early one morning with a long list of supplies needed for the hospital and for themselves. It was still early in the hyperinflation cycle, and although prices increased on a monthly basis, most items were still available in the stores. Before they left, I went to my secret hiding place to find some "bricks" of money—freshly minted "$10,000 promissory notes" in packets of 100. I placed 40 bricks in an old shopping bag, handed it to Sheila and said, "Take good care of this and don't spend it all in one place."

"How much is in here?" she asked.

"Oh, only 40 million."

"But how much is it *really?*"

"At the latest rate, it's about U.S. $400. It takes ten of the $10,000 notes to make a dollar."

"Wow."

They needed most of it because the hospital supplies came to over $300 and their personal shopping was another $90. With each passing month, we needed larger and larger bags to carry the bricks of money needed to buy the same amount of supplies. A year later, when I needed two new tires for the car, I carried a large cardboard box full of bricks of $10,000 notes into the store, plunked it on the counter and said, "Here's five hundred million." It was barely enough for two tires. Soon after, the government changed currencies and printed even larger denominations as the inflation spiral zoomed into the stratosphere.

While the ladies were shopping in Masvingo, a tremendous thunderstorm came through, dropping two inches of rain in two hours. Loretta knew the "short-cut" road back home would probably be flooded, so she drove the extra 20 miles to take the safer road. As she approached the first of the low bridges on that road, a foot or more of water was flowing over it. Thoughts of returning from Kwe Kwe in 1975 flooded through her mind, and she knew they had to wait until the water receded.

"What do we do now?" asked Sheila.

"Wait for the water to go down."

"How long will that take?"

"Usually just an hour or so, but sometimes longer," and she proceeded to tell Sheila of her escapade when returning from Marist Brothers' School in 1975. That led to other adventures by the Stoughton Clan during the 1970's, and the time quickly passed. After waiting an hour, a low-slung Mazda pickup approached from the other direction and slowly made its way across the bridge, water flowing halfway up the wheels. Loretta said, "If he can make it across, so can we." Sheila prayed as Loretta cautiously inched her way across the bridge, both exhaling a sigh of relief as they reached the other side. There were three more underwater bridges to cross, and Loretta could hear Sheila mumbling 'Hail Mary's' as they edged across each one.

At least once or twice a week we joined the Cavanaugh's for dinner or to play cards or board games, and drink a beer—or two, or a glass of Zimbabwean or South African wine. Having the Cavanaugh's as friends helped to keep us mentally healthy and gave us a renewal of energy. Maybe our "health and energy" was going to last a few more years? The hole in the bottom of that water tank was at least temporarily plugged.

Not long after they arrived, Doctor Clara began making serious plans for starting a residency in O.B./GYN. Her first desire was to do it in South Africa because the training would be better than in Zimbabwe. There were good doctors to work under in Zimbabwe, but the situation in the country had steadily deteriorated since 2000, and supplies in the government hospitals were becoming more scarce with each passing month. She finally obtained the necessary financial backing and was accepted into a program at Witwatersrand University in Johannesburg, leaving St. Theresa's in October

2003. Once again there were just the two of us. *But remember, you're not alone, and you're lucky to have the Cavanaugh's.*

In early 2004, I was doing a physical exam on one of our new student nurses. Mrs. Murungu was a middle-aged woman who had been accepted into our nurses training program, and I began questioning her: how she came to be in the program—"I always wanted to be a nurse;" where she was from—"Rusape;" and whether she had children—"Yes, five of them. In fact, my son Joseph just finished his two-year Internship at Mpilo Hospital in Bulawayo, and thinks he might like to come to St. Theresa's." I learned that he had driven his mother to the nursing school, liked the way the hospital looked, thought it would be a good experience, and he needed a job. Long story short, he came for an interview and shortly afterwards started to work for us and stayed until after we left in 2009.

Dr. Joseph Murungu was a gem. Like Tim Cavanaugh, he was intelligent, hard working, soft-spoken, very caring with his patients, and easy to get along with. The three of us worked together like a well-oiled machine. I thought to myself, *"This is great. I could work for many more years in this environment. Thank you God."* Having three at the hospital gave us breathing room so that when one was away, there was still enough help to comfortably get the work done on a daily basis. It also allowed me to present them with a proposal: "Since I'm now 67, would it be okay if I stopped taking call?"

As I got older, it became more and more difficult to get back to sleep when I was called during the night. In fact, I usually would not get back to sleep at all and would be wiped out the next day. Early in our medical careers, doctors have to learn how to wake up in the middle of the night, be instantly alert to handle whatever emergency is at hand, and when the problem is over, quickly get back to sleep. Otherwise we wouldn't survive, and I prided myself on how good I was at doing that.

During my years in Wisconsin and while raising our big family, Loretta and I had an agreement: During the night, I would answer the phone and take care of the medical problems and she would take care of the middle-of-the-night kid problems. She didn't hear the phone ring and I didn't hear the kids cry. At times I would answer the phone, get out of bed, go to the hospital, and later get back into bed without her even knowing I was gone. It worked out well for us. We lived only a half-block from the hospital, and I used to kid with some of my O.B. patients that I could get to the hospital in one minute, be in the delivery room in two minutes, deliver their baby and be back home and in bed in five minutes, hardly waking up in the interval! Of course, that wasn't true but it made a good story.

Once I was called at 2:00 A.M. to the emergency room to see an elderly man from the Nursing Home. His son, a County Judge, was there with him. We knew each other well and I greeted him, "Hey, Tom. What's going on?"

With bleary eyes, he looked at me, shook his head and said, "How can you be so chipper when getting called in the middle of the night? I've been up for an hour and still can't get my eyes open."

"We learn it in Med School. It goes along with the job," I replied. "Now let's see what's wrong with your Dad."

Because Tim and Joseph had pity on the "old guy," they readily agreed to the arrangement. If one of them was away for more than a week, then I would take my turn on call, but otherwise the burden was removed.

In 2004 we also were able to slowly initiate our AIDS treatment program. Tim had experience treating AIDS patients in the Indian Health Service, and Joseph had some experience during his training, so between the three of us we were able to devise a small program, starting with some of our staff members who needed treatment. As described in the previous chapter, it slowly became a primary focus of the mission of our hospital.

After three wonderful years with the Cavanaugh's, they left at the end of 2006, having completed their contract with Mission Doctors Association. With tears in our eyes, we watched them go through the check-in process at Harare International Airport. There was no replacement, primarily because of the increasing political instability in the country and the worries MDA had about the safety of their doctors. (They knew we were staying, *almost no matter what.*) It was also becoming more and more difficult for expatriate doctors to get a medical license in Zimbabwe, for a myriad of bureaucratic reasons. With no help coming from Los Angeles, I began looking for another Zimbabwe doctor. I didn't have to look far because one day Joseph came to me and said a friend of his had just finished his internship and was looking for work. Dr. Changa was a nice guy, but he didn't have nearly the ethics, energy nor compassion for patients that Joseph did. Still, he was a good doctor and in most cases he did credible work.

In one instance, he didn't. On his own, he decided to do a hernia repair on 30-year-old Gerald. During the procedure, he sent an urgent call to me for help. He had gotten into some serious bleeding and didn't know what to do. When he started at St. Theresa's I told him he should *not* do any surgery other than C-sections, since he didn't have any formal training in surgery. Still, he thought he could do this "simple case." During my residency training, one of the surgeons said to me, "Remember this even if you don't remember anything else I teach you: There are no simple surgical cases, only simple surgeons."

I scrubbed and gowned and assessed the problem. He was deep into the left groin—way too low for repairing a hernia—and had gotten into the femoral vessels, the main blood supply to the leg. I didn't think he was in the femoral artery, but there was a lot of bleeding and it was difficult to tell where it was coming from. Maybe there was a small tear in the femoral vein, which would be just as serious. He had attempted to put sutures around the bleeding sites, but at least he knew enough to not use deep sutures, as they could cut off all the blood supply to the leg. I carefully isolated some of the small bleeders and tied them off. There was still a lot of oozing blood from deep within the wound. With pressure I was able to stop the bleeding, so I used pressure and waited fifteen minutes. It seemed to have stopped, but then started again. After two hours, I felt I finally had it under control, but was really worried about the leg. A bit of blood was still oozing. Could he have gotten the deep vessels? The leg was cool but not cold. There were pulses in the left foot, but not the same as in the right. I was worried.

"Damn, damn, damn, Dr. Changa. Didn't I tell you not to do cases unless I was with you? What were you thinking of?"

"I had watched these during internship. They looked simple, so I thought I wouldn't bother you."

"Well, you've certainly bothered me now. What are we going to do? I don't think we can keep him here with the possibility that he might lose his leg. You could lose your license if he does, and this hospital would be in trouble. He needs to see a vascular surgeon who can better assess the situation."

I discussed it with Dr. Murungu. My first choice was to take the man to nearby Driefontein, where Dr. Aschwanden would be able to handle it, but a telephone call informed us he was gone for the week. Dr. Murungu knew a vascular surgeon in Harare, so we made arrangements to take Gerald there. I didn't feel comfortable sending him in our ambulance without a doctor along, so I drove the ambulance myself, with Gerald and Dr. Murungu in the back, an I.V. running, and Dr. Murungu checking Gerald's blood pressure and making sure there was no new bleeding.

Our ambulance was only six-months old, the result of a generous donor in the U.S. I had driven it a few times, but not on a long trip. I was enjoying using the siren to have cars get out of my way, but halfway to Harare, as I accelerated on the outskirts of Chivhu, I had to slam on the brakes to avoid a donkey that ran directly in front of me. I still hit it with the right front fender, knocking it to the ground. It hee-hawed loudly a few times, bounded to its feet and ran off. I got out of the ambulance to inspect the damage. The right front light was broken, but everything else seemed to be okay. There was no obvious leaking of fluid and the vehicle drove alright, so we continued on our way. Thirty miles later, the temperature gauge started rising to near the boiling point. *Damn, damn, damn. What else can go wrong?*

Steam was coming from the radiator and I could see a tiny hole in the middle of it. Now what? We were in the middle of nowhere, had a patient who urgently needed help, and no nearby garage. Who can I call for help? One good piece of luck was that we were in an area where there was cell phone coverage—not very common out in the countryside. I was able to get in touch with Ed Sim, a good friend who owned some factories in Harare. I explained the situation and he arranged to send one of his workers with a vehicle that could tow us if necessary, but would also have several containers of water. Maybe the radiator had a slow enough leak that we could stop whenever it started to heat up, put in more water, and continue.

We impatiently waited two hours for the man to arrive. Fortunately, Gerald was fine, with no new bleeding and his leg remained the same. We filled the radiator and started for Harare, had to stop three times along the way to add more water, but made it safely. I dropped Dr. Murungu and Gerald off at the hospital, and proceeded to Emerald Hill for a restless nights sleep, still worried about Gerald's leg. The next process was to find a place to repair the ambulance. Ed was helpful for that also—he seemed to know everyone in Harare. Due to the lack of replacement parts it took several months for the repair and cost $2,500 U.S., but finally we had our "new" ambulance back in working order. The man did not lose his leg and was soon discharged from the hospital, but *without* the hernia being repaired. So much for a "simple surgical procedure."

I couldn't be too angry with Dr. Changa because I remembered that episode with the rivet in the lung of a small child in 1970, and in that situation, the child died. We all make wrong decisions, but some have worse outcomes. A banged up fender and radiator sure is better than a dead child. Dr. Changa promised not to do any more surgery unless I was there to assist.

STEP TWENTY-THREE

MIDDLE-OF-THE-NIGHT VISITORS

May 2006, 3:00 AM Sunday Morning: I woke with a start—did I hear a noise? No, probably just a dream. Our bedroom was at the rear of the house, with the toilet room nearby, and the bath and washbasin in a separate room across the hall. Leading to the front of the house was a long hallway with the kitchen and a small bedroom on the left, a storage room on the right, and at the end of the hall on the right was the door to the main living area. Since I was already awake, I got up to pee, flushed the toilet, walked to the lavatory room to wash my hands, looked down the hall and wondered why the door to the dining room was closed? We always left it open. I walked to the door and opened it to find the lights blazing in the dining and living rooms and the front door wide open. *Why did Loretta leave the door open? Was there some bad smell in the house so she decided to air it out?* As I walked into the living room it was obvious it wasn't Loretta who did this. A broken screen was lying on the floor, burglar bars on the outside of a window had been pried apart, papers and books were strewn everywhere. The drawers of my desk were turned upside down, and at first glance I could see that my laptop and back-up hard drive were missing. *Oh my God. What else is missing? Who did this?*

I woke Loretta and we walked into the living room. "What a mess. Do you think they just left?"

"I didn't hear them, but I think so."

"I'm glad you didn't walk in on them. You might have been hurt."

"I know. I wonder what's missing?"

247

"Let's look and see." We wandered around in a bit of a fugue state—picking up bits and pieces and putting them down and picking them up again, walking into a bedroom to see the clothes closet open and empty of clothes, commenting that "This is gone, that is gone, what do we do?"

I admitted to her, "When I first saw the open door, I thought 'Why did you leave the door open? Was there a bad smell in the house?' "

Haughtily she replied, "Just like a man. Blame it on the woman."

In a small storage room, more papers were on the floor. Tablecloths, bed sheets and pillowcases, my expensive camera, and a projector were missing. But, most importantly, the briefcase containing our passports and tickets for an upcoming vacation in South Africa, and Loretta's ticket to the States, was not to be found. (It was before the era of E-tickets, so we needed the actual paper tickets.)

"They must have heard me when I flushed the toilet and ran out the front door," I said.

"Let's see where they went."

With a flashlight, we cautiously walked out the front door to be greeted with a large hole in the bamboo fencing on the North side of our lawn and garden. I walked outside the fence and saw where they probably ran down a path towards the nearby township. There must have been two or three to carry the haul of so many items.

"What do we do now?"

"We need to report it to the Police." Since we had no external phone, at 3:30 AM I took the car out of our locked garage and drove to the nearby Police Camp. A night-duty woman officer took the information and told me someone would be at our house shortly. I returned home and the two of us made a list of missing items: two Dell laptop computers; back-up hard drive; Sony digital projector; Olympus digital camera with ten-x telephoto lens and carrying bag; briefcase with passports and airline tickets; two Nokia cell phones and chargers; baby clothes; bed sheets and pillow cases; some cash I had in the desk drawer; two Kenwood stereo speakers—total replacement value of $5,000. A cardboard box we used for storing woven baskets must have served as a convenient container for carting off the loot.

Two sleepy policemen came to take our statements and make a survey of the house. To me, they didn't seem very bright and *not* at all professional. No concern about fingerprints (maybe they didn't have the technology to collect them?), no "preserving the crime scene," no pictures taken—police work from the 70's. They only wrote down what we told them and didn't ask many questions. They looked at the hole in the fence and walked around to see where the thieves had fled the property, shook their heads and said, "Yes, it seems they went that way to the township." *No kidding, Sherlock Holmes. Good deductive reasoning.*

At 6:00 AM, the "Member in Charge" (Chief) Policeman arrived with some other officers. He was more professional, but of course the "crime scene" had been terribly contaminated by then, and he still didn't have the ability to take fingerprints, and still no camera. I took pictures with Loretta's small camera that was fortunately in our bedroom. *How I wish we had kept some of the other expensive items there.*

He asked me, "Do you have any suspicions? It looks like it could be someone who knows your house. What about your maid?"

"Never. I would trust Monica with everything we have."

"Anyone else?"

"Not that I can think of. There are many people who work at the hospital who have a good idea of the layout of this house, but I wouldn't want to accuse anyone."

"Let me know if you think of someone. We'll find them, I promise you. Make a detailed list of all missing items and bring that to the station. We'll file a report and start the investigation."

As the police continued to poke here and there looking for clues, I fixed fresh coffee for everyone and told Loretta to get ready for 7:00 AM Mass. She could talk with the priest before Mass, tell him what happened, ask him to announce the burglary and plead with the people to ask for the return of our passports and tickets. I did the same before the 9:00 AM Mass. We did think this was most likely an "inside job" by someone from the area—someone who knew our house quite well—and maybe through the "bush telegraph" they would hear of our request.

Before he left, the police chief and I walked down the path that led to the township. About 300 yards down the path, carelessly thrown into a thorn bush, was my briefcase. I rushed to pick it up, hoping against hope to find the passports and airline tickets. No such luck. It was empty. *Why the briefcase but not the tickets and passports? Now we'll have to go to the U.S. Embassy in Harare for new passports and to South African Airlines for replacement tickets. I wonder how long that will take? Can we get new passports before we're supposed to leave for South Africa? Darn!*

For the rest of that day a continuous stream of people came to offer their condolences and support. It was almost as if someone had died. A common comment was, "How could anyone do that to you? After all the good the two of you have done. We're so sorry. Is there anything we can do to help?" One of the Sisters brought a casserole so Loretta wouldn't have to cook that day.

Tim and Sheila came to give us support. Tim lamented with me on the loss of the backup hard-drive that had so much information on it, and now everything that was on my computer would be gone forever. "I wouldn't have done anything different than you did. It's important to backup the computer, but I never would have worried about burglars. Now I will."

No one could believe the burglars had the audacity to break into the house *while we were in the house sleeping*! How could they do that? One woman said, "You know, they have some sort of magical potion they spray in the house and it causes you to remain asleep." The African suspicion of witchcraft remains strong.

"No, I don't think so," I answered. "2:00 AM is when you're in the deepest sleep, so it takes a lot of noise to wake you. I think I must have finally heard something, and that's what woke me at 3:00."

Ms. Hove, our administrator, lived next door to us and came to survey the scene. "I think it was someone we know and who knows your house," she said. "You know, Sydney Murume who was working in Admin, left without notice two weeks ago and hasn't returned. I heard he was in the Township last night. One of the student nurses is his girlfriend, even though he has a wife and family in Harare." Sydney had been recommended to us by one of the government officials in the Mission Section of the Ministry of Health. He was quite good with computers, and seemed to pick up the admin work quickly—too quickly, it turned out.

"That's possible. He came to the house recently to get my signature on a check. I sat at our dining room table to sign it, so he would have known the set-up of our house. It seems the thieves knew exactly where to look for the expensive items. We both feel violated with them breaking into our house while we were sleeping. When I got up to use the bathroom, I think they heard the toilet flush and ran out the front door. Maybe that's lucky, because I wouldn't have wanted to surprise them inside the house. If I did, something worse might have happened to me."

Early Monday morning, Nikolas our gardener knocked on the door. "Doctor, I found these over near the corner of the fence." He handed me two passports and three airline tickets! Apparently the announcement in church worked. The burglars felt a bit of compassion for us and when they realized the tickets and passports had no value to them (might even be dangerous), they must have returned in the middle of the night and thrown them over the fence. Thank God for small favors. Wish I had asked for the backup hard drive too. At least we wouldn't have to go through the pain of replacing the passports and getting new tickets. We could still go for that holiday in South Africa the next week. We needed a vacation to recover from this invasion of our privacy.

Since I was going to need a new laptop and camera, at the last minute I changed my plans and accompanied Loretta on her visit to the States. She already had a ticket to leave the day after we returned from South Africa, so it was good timing for me to take the opportunity to fly with her, see all the kids and grandkids, and get the new equipment I needed. *Every cloud has a silver lining.* A second silver lining was when I reported the burglary to my insurance agent: I found that since I had "renters insurance" to cover the boxes we had stored at our son's house, the insurance covered burglary, even in Zimbabwe. With a copy of the police report, I was reimbursed for replacement costs after a $200 deductible. What a nice surprise. Everything was replaced—except the data on my computer. I thought I was smart to have a backup hard drive that I faithfully used every month, but it was to protect data if my computer crashed, and not from a burglary—especially since I had the backup right next to the laptop. If only I had kept the backup next to my bed. All that information lost, but the worst was the pictures that would never be viewed again. *Well, no one died or was injured. We felt "violated" but would get over that. There was such an outpouring of support from everyone in the community. It made us feel special and loved. We got our passports and tickets back, had a nice vacation in South Africa and even a better one in the U.S.* We "locked the door after the horse was gone" by installing a security alarm that would frighten anyone trying to break into the house and awaken the entire neighborhood.

When we returned from our vacation, there was a message the police chief wanted to see me. After walking the half-mile to the station, I was greeted by the Member in Charge. "Hello doctor. How are you?"

"Fine, how are you?"

"Fine. I have some news about the Mr. Murume. Maybe you heard that he used a stolen hospital check that already had two signatures on it to buy a fridge in Mashava?

"Yes, Ms Hove told me about that. We've already made policy changes on how we sign checks."

"Then last week, one of my officers was in Masvingo and saw him walking on the other side of the street. He was carrying two small boxes. She wanted to question him, but he recognized her as she crossed the street, dropped the boxes and ran. The boxes had medicines from the National Pharmacy and a copy of a St. Theresa Hospital request form."

"So he also stole some request forms. Too bad he got away. Now what?"

"We now know for sure that he was the one who broke into your house, and now these two additional crimes. We'll get him."

"I hope so. Maybe he'll still have my backup hard-drive."

Even though the police were good at tracking down political foes, Sydney was never apprehended. We suspected someone was protecting him from high up in government—maybe the same one who recommended him to us? Or maybe my paranoia was just running amuck.

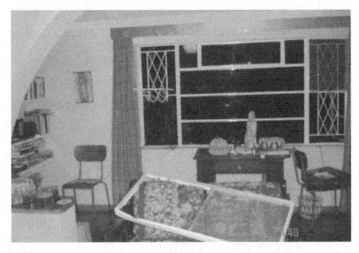

Living room after the robbery - window bars were bent up where they got in

VISITING A RURAL
ZIMBABWE FAMILY

S ister Letwina, a charismatic African Sister with a quick wit and engaging
smile, was student teaching at the Mission primary school. She was a
lot of fun to be around and immensely popular with the children. She and
Loretta became good friends, so when she came to us saying she needed help
with her tuition fees for her last year at the Teachers College, we agreed to
help. Once she had a teaching certificate, her salary would be a financial boon
for her congregation. We felt it was a good investment, under the heading:
"Give a woman a fish and you feed her for a day; teach her to fish, and you
feed her for a lifetime."

Just before she returned to college, she invited us to visit her family
home near Berejena Mission. Jumping at the chance for such an adventure,
one Saturday in late March we drove two hours South of St. Theresa's to pick
her up, along with a companion, Sister Georgina. We drove 60 miles on the
main road towards South Africa—familiar to us because of our frequent
trips across the border for shopping—before turning onto the dirt road
towards Berejena Mission—one of the clinics I flew to in the 1970's. The
sandy road was better than ours because there were neither deep gorges to
maneuver the Isuzu down, nor rivers to cross. To say the road was dusty
was an understatement. It was the end of the rainy season and once again
there had been little rain. The few maize stalks looked like lonely sentinels
drooping in the mid-day heat. I doubt if any maize was harvested that year.
As we drove, we passed mammoth granite outcroppings. They stood out on
the otherwise flat barren land looking like multiple huge football stadiums

scattered higgledy-piggledy, as if some Giant had angrily strewn them about. After 1½ hours, we turned left, and soon arrived at Sisters' "homestead"—an oasis in the midst of the desert-like surroundings.

It was impressive, to say the least: Four large nicely constructed cement block homes with normal asbestos-sheet roofing graced the fenced compound. Upon entering, we were greeted by three large barking dogs that quickly sensed we were not intruders, and then by Sisters' mother, grandmother, a brother and his wife and children, plus many other women and children. I later learned the "others" were the widows and children of Sisters' three deceased brothers, a typical "rural African extended family." I didn't count them, but there must have been at least twenty people. Greetings abounded and we were shown around the compound: an outdoor cooking area with heavy poles on the corners and covered with a thatched roof; their own shallow well with a turning handle and bucket; a generator fueled with diesel—but none available at the time; two outdoor pit toilets, one for the men and one for the women; a separate shower area with water in a large bucket on the roof; three graves covered with flat, black soapstone, marking the three brothers graves; several round traditional African style huts plus the four rectangular-shaped houses, each with their own dining room, living room, and bedrooms.

Sister Letwina took us into the house where we would sleep. The door entered into a dining room with a beautiful wooden dining table and chairs. Next was a living room with overstuffed couches and chairs, and a bedroom furnished with a double bed and a thick mattress and box springs. Loretta almost had to jump to sit on the bed. After leaving our small travel bag, we went outside to sit and talk with Sisters' family. From the size and quality of the homestead, we could see that someone must have a good job for them to afford such a nice place.

"You have a lovely homestead," I said to Samuel, Sister's oldest brother.

"Thank you. We have worked hard to make it this way," he replied, exuding an air of competence as we sat and talked.

"Someone must have a good job in town to be able to afford these houses."

"Yes, all my brothers had good jobs, but now three of them have died within the past seven years." I didn't ask, but from what Sister told me, I surmised they had died from AIDS.

"What do you do, Samuel?"

"I own an acreage near Kyle Lake where I irrigate thirty acres. It's good land, and with irrigation I can grow two or three crops every year. The maize was excellent this year, and now I've planted beans for the early winter season and will try winter wheat later."

"That's a lot of work."

"It is, but I love it. I have three young men working for me. We do all the work by hand, so it keeps us busy. I seldom get home, but I wanted to be here when you came with Letwina. I'm the senior male for the compound, and it would be impolite for me to be away."

"Loretta and I thank you for the invitation." Nodding at the generator I said, "What do you use it for?"

"We don't use it much. It's just for lights, but with diesel so expensive and difficult to get, its not worth it. We're used to not having lights at night. We just go to bed early and get up at dawn."

"Who takes care of all of this?" I asked, sweeping my hand around the large compound.

"My mother is in charge and she's good at managing my wife and all my sisters-in-law and their children to see that everything gets done."

"It doesn't look like there was much rain this year."

"Just like most years, so we have to grow drought resistant maize, and we also grow cotton that thrives in this hot environment. That's our biggest cash crop. But it's the irrigation scheme at Kyle that keeps us going."

"I saw all the cotton piled on one of the porches. What do you do with it?"

"The women hand-sort it into grades of cotton, pack it in those large burlap bags, and I sell it at the Grain Marketing Board."

"Could you show me your garden?" We walked through a meticulously planted and cultivated garden of beans, spinach, kale, cabbage, tomatoes, onions, and a few rows of maize. There were orange, avocado, lemon, papaya, and banana trees. It really looked like an oasis. "Do you irrigate all this?"

"Yes, the women and children draw water from the well and bring it one bucket at a time to carefully water each plant and tree. We use cow manure from the kraal for fertilizer."

"It's beautiful. I have running water for our small garden plus a gardener, and it doesn't look as nice as yours."

Within the compound chickens ran here and there, clucking and pecking at seeds and insects. Outside the fence, many goats were roaming freely amid a herd of thirty cattle that were being watched by a young boy with a homemade whip. He enjoyed using it to make a loud cracking noise—not hitting the beasts, but making a loud snap so everyone knew he was doing his job.

"Are the goats and cattle all yours?" I asked Samuel.

"Yah. We try to limit the number of goats. As you know, we Africans count our wealth by the number of cattle we own, so we try to maintain a healthy herd. It's not easy in years when there's so little grass for grazing. I bring some of the corn stalks from my land at Kyle, so that helps."

Loretta was talking with Sister and some of the women, and eventually they were all sitting on the porch where the Ambuya—grandmother—was sorting cotton. With a deeply wrinkled face, she looked to be in her 80's, but it's difficult to tell an African's age because long days working in the sun causes premature aging of the skin. She had just a few snags for teeth but a beautiful smile. She didn't speak any English, so Sister translated.

"Ambuya, how do you sort the cotton?" Loretta asked.

The Ambuya proceeded to show her how to see what the color was, how to feel the quality of the cotton ball, and how the seeds felt. She would take each cotton ball, finger it, remove the seed and then sort it into three piles: Grade One—no bits of leaf or stem and pure white color (the best); Grade Two—some bits of stem and perhaps a yellow stain; or Grade Three— all the rest. Each pile would then be placed in large burlap bags and labeled with the grade.

Soon all the women, Loretta included, were sitting on the cement porch sorting cotton and picking out the seeds. It might have been a scene from our antebellum South except for the one white woman sitting there talking and joking with the others, even if she didn't understand much that was being said.

Walking around the compound, it was obvious there were many differences from our own "compound" at St. Theresa's. We had a similarly shaped house and a large garden and our area was fenced, but we had electricity (most of the time), clean running water, and an indoor toilet. The other striking difference was that we had a nice lawn and here there was no grass. I felt a sense of calmness when I sat on our verandah at the end of a long and trying day and gazed at our green lawn. No rural African would waste time or energy on grass when they could use the same time and energy on a garden. Here, everything not garden was bare dirt, pounded firm by bare feet incessantly walking over every square inch. The first thing each morning, the young girls used homemade brooms and bending over at the waist, quickly swept the entire area until it looked as if it had been vacuumed, all the while chatting and giggling and casting furtive glances at the visitors.

During the rainy season it must have been muddy and uncomfortable, but it hadn't rained for weeks, so no mud—just cleanly swept hard-packed dirt.

Towards the end of the day, we could hear the cattle being driving to a pen near the compound. The "cattle kraal," a small area fenced with wooden poles, kept them corralled for the night and prevented them from wandering into gardens and planted fields. During the night we would hear the cattle complaining when one of the others would bump against them, or maybe just letting us know they were having a bad dream. Who knows what cattle think?

It was getting late and time for the evening meal. I had hoped we would sit around and eat with all of the other people in the compound, but no, that would not be polite. Sister came to us and said, "It's time to eat. Let's go into the house and sit."

"But Sister, I'd really like to eat with the rest of your relatives."

"Oh no, they would not want you to do that. You are our guests, so you must eat at the dining table that is already set."

Sisters Letwina and Georgina joined Loretta and me as the lone diners at the large table. Young girls came with platters of fried chicken, sadza, rice, and vegetables. We were offered either Coca Cola or Fanta Orange, and later had tea. Our conversations were subdued, but we heard raucous laughing from outside and again I wished we could have joined those people, but it wouldn't have been polite in their culture. After eating, we joined the rest of the family. I had my laptop computer to show some pictures of wild animals, and then I showed a short Roadrunner cartoon movie. I had the children sit near the computer while I stood behind. They jabbered excitedly in Shona about the wonders they were witnessing. Screeches and shouts of laughter filled the air, some of it by the adults who enjoyed it nearly as much, but they especially delighted in the reactions of their young children. Our grand-children are so used to T.V., movies, videos, and game-boys that what I was showing would be dull to them, but these children had never seen such a thing before and were enthralled.

It was time for bed, so Loretta and I each visited the appropriate pit toilet, using the flashlights we brought, and then said goodnight to all. There were candles in our bedroom, we crawled into bed, blew out the candle and kissed goodnight. "It was a lovely evening," she said.

"Yes it was," and I was quickly asleep. It seemed like just a few minutes later when Loretta nudged me and said, "Dick, wake up. I have to use the toilet."

I looked at my watch—three A.M. I couldn't believe I had slept so long and so soundly. I lit the candle, found our flashlights, and we carefully walked out the front door, only to be greeted with loud barking from all three dogs. Loudly whispering I tried to get the dogs to "shush," but to no avail. Finally someone from one of the other houses *shouted* at the dogs and they stopped barking, but not before everyone in the compound was awake. We walked to the toilet, and by that time, every door on the compound was open with dark faces peering out. I shrugged my shoulders and hoped they understood. Loretta went inside with her flashlight, squatted down over the hole in the floor, and finished. She whispered to me as we walked back to our bed, "So much for quietly using the bathroom in the middle of the night."

The next day was Sunday, and we all planned on going to Mass at a small church three miles away. After a breakfast of porridge and bread, we washed ourselves in the shower area and dressed for church. It was supposed to start at 10:00, but true to African custom, it finally began at 10:30. Time is really of no meaning to people who use the sun to tell time; it is only us who think schedules are important who want things to "be on time." Of course, we are the ones dying of heart attacks.

As we walked towards the church, people came from all directions to greet Sister Letwina. Such joy for them to see this young woman they had known since childhood, looking so elegant in her smart-looking Nun's outfit. Everyone knew everyone, and church on Sunday was an opportunity to catch up on local gossip both before and after the service. Drumming from inside the church indicated that Mass would soon begin. It was all in Shona, but I knew enough to understand the prayers and songs. The deep basso male voices blended beautifully with the soprano of the women and the sound reverberated through the small church and into the countryside. The "Gloria" really did sound glorious, with the Shona words for "Glory to God in the Highest" sung over and over in such wondrous praise and glory. I thought, *African people know how to sing in church. I wish we had this in our churches at home. I guess many of the Black churches do.* The songs were accompanied by drums and the blowing of a Kudu horn, and at intervals by an old Ambuya ululating—yeeyeeyeeyee, in a varying high-pitched shout. I could see some of the younger people smirking about the shouting, but no one would ever castigate an Ambuya for doing it.

After gossiping for a half hour after Mass, we returned to Sister's home to collect our luggage and say our goodbyes. Sister Letwina and Sister Georgina were staying a few days, so after thanking everyone, we climbed into the car and slowly exited the gate, with dogs barking and people waving goodbye. Small boys and dogs ran as fast as they could to follow us to the turn in the road.

ELECTIONS

Saturday Morning, March 29, 2008: We were walking to the Mission for 7:00 A.M. Mass. The sun was poking its nose over the Eastern hills, roosters were crowing, and birds were raucously greeting the new day. Something different was in the air. People were streaming towards the Mission from all compass points, a newfound bounce in their step, faces adorned with smiles, greetings shouted back and forth, waves and high-fives abounding. One might think they were on their way to a World Cup Soccer match, but no, it was Election Day 2008.

For once it appeared the elections were going to be peaceful, so instead of fleeing the country, Loretta and I stayed at St. Theresa's. Previously, we made sure we were out of Zimbabwe leading up to any voting because of the expected and usual violence. This time, many Zimbabweans were hoping and praying for a change in leadership. Robert Mugabe was the only leader the country had known since Independence in 1980. He ruled with an iron fist and tolerated no disagreement within his ZANU-PF political party *or* from any opposition. There even were laws on the books making it a serious offense to make *any* disparaging remarks about the aging ruler. He was 84, and there were rumors he was in failing health—but those hope-filled rumors had been circulating for years, and he still appeared fit and robust.

A viable opposition party—The Movement for Democratic Change, or MDC—had arisen, with Morgan Tsvangarai (Chang´-grr-aye´) at the helm. He was a Trade Union organizer, and people were hoping he might be the "Lech Walesa" of Zimbabwe—the Trade Unionist who transformed Poland from Communism to a thriving post-communist economy in the 1990's.

They hoped a new face and new policies might do the same for Zimbabwe. Others remained faithful to "The Old Man" and wanted him to continue as their leader.

*

To understand rural politics in Zimbabwe, one must first understand the system of "Tribal Chiefs." For centuries, Chiefs were the local leaders, and traditionally that leadership role was passed down within the same family. Early on, the Colonial powers recognized that continuing the power of the Chief was a way for them to control the rural people. If they paid—or bribed—the Chiefs, then the Chiefs would do as the government demanded, and thus the Chiefdom system continued throughout Colonial Africa. The rural people were accustomed to having a Chief and strongly supported him. In its best use, it's a good system. The Chief and his Sub-chiefs and Counselors settle small—and a few big—disputes so they don't clog up the police or court system. Many Chiefs are genuinely concerned about the welfare of their subjects, but like any system where there is power, abuse easily creeps into the equation. There is no way to eliminate a bad Chief—except by murder or natural death. He is only replaced when he dies, and then another of his family becomes the new Chief and might be just as evil as the old one. Rural Zimbabweans couldn't perceive of a system where Chiefs would be elected— it wasn't part of their culture and tradition.

Mugabe grew up in rural Rhodesia and was well acquainted with the importance of the Chief. After coming to power, he continued most of the oppressive laws the Whites had used to control the Blacks, but now he used them to control any and all opposition, but most importantly, any Black opposition. He also continued the Colonialist custom of paying—bribing— the Chiefs so he could maintain control over them. Even as overwhelming opposition developed in the urban centers, his popularity in most rural areas remained firm. I say "most" because he had little support in Matabeleland, the Southwest quarter of the country, where the predominant tribe is Ndebele.

During the 1980's, Mugabe violently destroyed an insurrection and opposition party that was based in rural Matabeleland. During that internal conflict, both sides committed murders and atrocities. Turmoil and uncertainty was rampant in the struggling, newly independent country. The Fifth Brigade of the Army, after being trained by the vicious North Koreans, was sent by Mugabe to end the insurrection. They did it by savagely murdering more than 20,000 men, women, and children. To stop the bloodshed, Ndebele leader Joshua Nkomo signed a "Unity Accord" in 1987, effectively forcing the entire Matabeleland Province into a newly formed political party, Zimbabwe African National Union-Patriotic Front (ZANU-PF).[4] With Mugabe's history in Matabeleland, most Ndebele's had little love for him.

It soon became traditional that before a national election, each Chief would suddenly receive a new four-wheel drive vehicle plus additional money, ostensibly to enable him to travel throughout his district so he could keep in close personal contact with his subjects. In actual fact, it was so he could travel to intimidate his people and make sure they continued to vote for ZANU-PF. Very few Chiefs in the country turned down this handout. Close to 100% supported Mugabe and his party.

St. Theresa Hospital was in the Chirumanzu District, and the people had always been overwhelmingly supportive of Mugabe. They looked upon him as their "Senior Chief"—likening him to a kindly old grandfather who would look after them and would always have their best interests at heart. However, much of that support and adoration of "The Old Man" was waning because of the severe hyperinflation, an unemployment rate of 90%, a chaotic and broken educational system, a medical system without proper medicines or supplies, and the absence of even the most basic items like corn meal and cooking oil in the local stores.

---

4   This atrocity is well documented in many books and articles—see Wikipedia for "Gukurundi Massacres."

*

As we walked to church that Saturday morning, we saw smiles instead of those gloomy looks that were so prominent because of the economic situation. It seemed that people were ready for a change and they thought this time it would finally happen. It was perhaps the fairest election in Zimbabwe in years, if not decades. At the end of the voting day, members from each party were on hand to supervise the tallying of votes, and the results were posted outside each voting precinct.

After the polls closed, I walked to the polling station at the Secondary School with other hospital employees. As we stood waiting in the evening twilight, an official came and tacked the results on the door: Mugabe 55%; Tsvangarai 45%. A few cheers; many groans; much mumbling.

"How could they still vote for the Old Man?"

"He bribes them with maize-meal and cooking oil, and they forget that within a month of the election, it's back to the same old thing—no food, no money, no jobs."

"Still, this is the best any opposition has ever done here. I think it means MDC wins, because they'll win big in the cities."

Soon there were choruses of "Yes, yes. We will win and there will be change." The mood quickly shifted from despair to triumph.

People were taking cell phone photos of the results and sending them to MDC headquarters in Harare. By using those photos from throughout the country, within two days the MDC was certain that Tsvangarai had won, and by a large margin—perhaps by as much as 65%. But they hadn't reckoned with the voting manipulation of Mugabe's party. It was even rumored that Mugabe was ready to concede defeat, but the Bigwigs in his party wouldn't let him. No results were forthcoming for a week, and then for two weeks, and then for a month. Finally the Electoral Commission (controlled by Mugabe and his ZANU-PF party) announced that Tsvangarai had 47.9% and Mugabe

43.2% of the vote, with the rest going to a minor candidate. Because no one had over 50% of the vote, there would have to be a run-off election.

The Army, Police, and C.I.O. (think KGB) were furious with the voters that they could vote for anyone other than their beloved leader, and they began a program of violence and intimidation, even before any "official" results were released. They knew Mugabe had lost and they were angry. Ann, a friend of ours from the U.S., was visiting at the time and was scheduled to leave in two weeks. Within a few days of the election, rumors began popping up at the hospital that caused me to be concerned about our safety. Sister Andrea took me aside one day and said, "There are rumors in the Township that you advised staff members to vote MDC, and even had staff meetings to encourage them."

"You know that's not true,"

"Yes, I know it, but I'm worried about you and Loretta. There's even talk of violence to our staff, and that could mean you."

"What should we do?"

"Maybe you should leave the country until this is over?"

"I'll think about it." I went home to discuss it with Loretta and Ann. There wasn't imminent danger, but I didn't want to wait until the last minute and then have trouble getting out of the country—or something worse. I called Harare and talked with Sister Patricia, who had her ear to the ground and could give me good advice.

After telling her about the local rumors, I said, "What should we do, Sister Patricia?"

"You should leave. There's going to be a lot of violence and no one can guarantee your safety."

We packed our bags, drove to the South African Airways in Harare, changed Ann's ticket, and purchased one-way tickets for us to Orlando where we could stay with our son Pete. We waited out the sham election of Mugabe in late June.

Tsvangarai eventually pulled out of that election because so many of his supporters were being brutalized and killed. The rest of the world didn't recognize the election results, and the country continued to dissolve into deeper and deeper chaos. Under pressure from neighboring African countries, a "Government of National Unity" (GNU) was eventually formed. GNU is an interesting acronym, since a Gnu (or Wildebeest) is an ungainly animal with large forefront and small hindquarters and scraggly whiskers—an ugly beast. The GNU proved to live up to its homonym.

Finally, at the end of August we returned to a relatively quiet Zimbabwe, but one that continued to be mired in the morass of hyper-hyperinflation, corruption at the highest levels, inefficiency at all levels of government, and an economy that was officially "in the tank." Gross Domestic Product had decreased by more than 50% since 2000. There was no hope for improvement in the foreseeable future because the newly elected government had no legitimacy and no new ways to deal with the overwhelming problems. The GNU was still in the making. The illegally elected Mugabe regime continued with the same old failing economic policies.

The most difficult problem was the horrible hyperinflation, which skyrocketed during the year. In January 2008, the *monthly* inflation rate was 120%—that meant that a loaf of bread that cost 100 *million* Zimbabwe dollars on the 1st of the month was 220 *million* by the end of the month. But the worst was yet to come. After we returned in late August, the September monthly inflation was 12,400%. Let's try to put that into perspective: For the third time, a new currency had been printed, with one million old dollars being worth one new dollar, but they immediately printed bills of a hundred million, a hundred billion, and later a hundred trillion dollars. That same loaf of bread that cost 220 million at the end of January, in the "new-Zim Dollars" was 22.4 *billion*, or if you add back the six zeros that had been deleted, 22.4

quadrillion dollars. You needed a wheelbarrow to carry enough money for grocery shopping.

A joke going around at the time of the new currency: Imagine an old, old wrinkled hunched-over Ambuya—grandmother—in a long line outside a bank, pushing her wheelbarrow full of "old dollars" to turn in for new ones. The line was moving slowly, and she urgently had to relieve herself. She turned to the man behind her and said, "Will you watch my money?" He agreed to do so. Returning 10 minutes later, she found her large pile of money but the wheelbarrow was gone!

There wasn't enough Zimbabwe currency to keep up with the demand, so all transactions soon occurred only on a barter basis *or* on the black market using foreign currency, especially U.S. dollars (called "yusas"). It was illegal to trade in yusas, but everyone—even the police—were doing it.

But it had not reached bottom yet. By November, the monthly inflation rate was 80 *billion* percent. I can't even attempt to give an example of how that translates into buying-power. Suffice it to say that no one had access to cash. People couldn't retrieve salaries that were directly deposited to their bank accounts. The only way for transactions to occur was through "inter-bank transfers" and writing personal checks, which no one—except maybe the Customs Agents at the borders—would accept. In December I was able to get trillions of dollars transferred into my account for an upcoming trip to South Africa.

With no commodities available in the local stores, the only way people survived was to make frequent trips to countries bordering Zimbabwe— countries where those same commodities were available in abundance. Shopkeepers in towns across the border were delighted to see the hordes of Zimbabwe shoppers. "Cross-border-trading" became a new occupation for those with valid passports. They crossed the borders to buy items at the limit allowed duty-free each month, brought them back to Zimbabwe, and sold them at a 50 to 100% profit—but sold them only in "yusas." Buses and trucks and cars were packed with Zimbabweans crossing the border for shopping. Customs Agents were busy day and night, and "brokers" who helped the traders through Customs—for a fee that was split with the Customs Agent—flourished.

After much negotiating, an agreement to include ZANU-PF, MDC-T, and MDC-M into the Government of National Unity was reached on September 15, 2008. Because of difficulty in working out the way this government would function, it wasn't formalized until February 11, 2009—amidst much hype, international television coverage, political speeches *ad nauseum*, and the typical politicians promise of a better tomorrow. At the same time, the GNU agreed to abandon the Zimbabwe currency and have a complete dollarization of the economy. Hyperinflation came to a screeching halt. Tendai Biti, the new Finance Minister, told everyone in government, "We can only eat what we kill," meaning that the government could no longer print money and had to live with the amount of tax revenues it collected. Such a novel idea—spend only what you have!

Although dysfunctional, the GNU did bring some economic growth to the country. But the police, army, and C.I.O remained under control of ZANU-PF, so false arrests, illegal incarcerations, and trumped-up charges not only continued but increased. To be in opposition to Mugabe meant you were his enemy and he would track you down and imprison you. After five years of this ugly beast of government, on July 31st, 2013 another election was held. This time the 89-year-old Mugabe had the entire vote-rigging machinery finely tuned, and he was once again re-elected—through massive voter fraud. The voter's role had over 100,000 people *over the age of 100!*—this in a country that had one of the lowest life expectancies in the world. Teenagers, too young to vote, were transported into cities and allowed to vote. Thousands of legitimate voters found their names were not on the voter list when they arrived at their normal polling place. The Southern African Development Community sent authorities to supervise, but they turned a blind eye and called the election "credible and fair." In a pig's eye it was. Mugabe apparently is convinced that he's the *only one* who can lead the impoverished nation. *Cry The Beloved Country.*

EMPTY SHELVES, FULL SHELVES

November 2008: I drove our Isuzu double-cab pickup over the 17 miles of sandy, bumpy road, up and down the steep embankments, and across the cement "underwater bridges." The road was impossible to navigate during the worst storms, and it was not unusual to have to wait on one side of such a bridge until the water went down enough to allow you to cross. Finally I was on the main road. Thirty miles of blacktop road, dotted with deep potholes that could easily cause you to overturn if hit at a high rate of speed.

Even though Masvingo had a population of 25,000, it was still very much a small town. Hyper-hyperinflation had caused money to become worthless. The government was printing 100 billion dollar "Promisory Notes"—we were all billionaires, but felt like paupers. Each note was initially worth $100 U.S., but after just a few weeks, it was worth only $1. I heard they would soon be printing $100 Trillion dollar notes. I hoped to get one just for a keepsake to show family and friends in the U.S. [5]

We had been shopping in Masvingo for years, and were hoping to get at least a few grocery supplies for ourselves and some items for the hospital—like toilet paper, soap, and cleaning supplies. As I walked into the warehouse grocery store—think of a very old, decrepit Sam's Club—I saw empty metal shelves, stretching into the distance like so many silent racks waiting for a miracle to happen. Here and there was a box of cookies or a tin of sardines, or a single wool sock that had lost its mate. It looked like a place that had already gone out of business. This sorry state of affairs happened because a few months previously, the government decided they would establish price

---

5   St. Theresa Hospital Annual Report 2008: Hyper-hyper inflation: in July it was 230 million percent; in August, 470 **billion** percent; in November, 90 **heptillion** percent (that's 90 followed by 21 zeroes).

controls on all goods. Then to be sure retail companies were totally ruined, they decreed that prices had to be rolled back to what they had been two months previously. In a hyperinflationary environment, that meant all items in every store were being sold at ridiculously low prices. Those fortunate few with access to Zimbabwe dollars via the Black Market could buy flat screen TVs for just a few U.S. dollars. All the shops were not only quickly out of everything, but also out of business—they had to sell items at a fraction of what they actually cost.

The higher-ups in government, who must have been forewarned about the event, were poised like vultures to swoop down upon the large retailers. They scoffed up the bargains into their greedy hands and drove away with trailers full of what they believed were their hard-won treasures—but were actually ill-gotten gains and downright thievery. Leading the crooks were Army Generals and Colonels, senior politicians, upper level policemen and women, and spouses of them all. Photos in the underground press looked like they were at some gala event, huge smiles on their faces, and captions of *"finally we took it to those wealthy capitalists."* Of course, it was just one more nail in the coffin of a dying Zimbabwe economy.

Now there was nothing to buy at the warehouse store, and it would most likely soon be out of business. I walked to another store that had a few items. "How can you get supplies?" I asked.

"Only because I'm selling in dollars or Rand."

"Is that legal?"

The owner shrugged his shoulders. I walked down the aisle to get a few of the absolutely necessary items: three rolls of toilet paper; one pound of margarine; one pound of salt; one quart of cooking oil. We were going to South Africa in a few weeks and could buy all we needed at a third the cost, but a few items we needed urgently. Looking furtively about for any secret police, I paid in dollars, and was out the door feeling like *I* might be the thief. *Is this the way normally law-abiding citizens become breakers of the law? Such a slippery slope. Of course, whenever we returned to Zimbabwe from South Africa we broke even more laws. I was becoming a real desperado.*

*

Next I went to the Police Station to visit the vehicle department. Before taking a vehicle to South Africa, I needed a permit to take it out of the country and then re-enter. It was a process that had to be repeated each time we went—just one more burdensome regulation making things difficult for the ordinary person. I filled out the requisite forms, produced the title, insurance papers, and authorizations from the Dominican Sisters saying I could take the car to South Africa, gave them all to the clerk, and said, "How long before I can pick up the permit?"

"Two hours at least," he mumbled without looking up. He could have done it right then, but like most civil servants in Zimbabwe, he had no motivation to really "serve" the people. Maybe he was waiting for a bribe? No matter how long I had to wait, I wasn't going to do that right in the middle of the police station. I didn't want to spend even a minute in a Zimbabwe jail.

It gave me time to go to a small outdoor café for lunch. Studio-52 was owned and operated by an ex-farmer and his wife who had lost their property during the takeover of white owned farms by the government in 2002 and 2003. Being a third generation family on the home farm, he really didn't know how to do anything except farming. Fortunately, he liked to cook— not gourmet, but plain, tasty, and filling. He and his artist wife were barely surviving by running the café, plus the little income from the few paintings she sold to the occasional tourist.

"Hey, Tom. How you doing today?"

"Just getting by, just getting by," he replied. He looked like a man who had been stretched on the rack and left to die alongside the road. Still, he also was optimistic, because he believed—hoped?—that something better was just around the corner. His was the sense of optimism that existed in the few white people who remained in Zimbabwe. Or maybe those still in the country really didn't have any place to go?

"What's on the menu today, Tom?"

"The usual. Hamburger and fries. Chicken. A bit of fish. What would you like?"

"I'll have the burger and fries, and some tea."

When it was time to pay, I asked him how much. "Do you have *yusas*?"

"Yeah."

"Then it's two dollars."

"That's not enough, Tom."

"I know, but it's what *they* say I have to charge."

I gave him three dollars, and went to a gas station to fill my pickup with diesel. Sounds like an easy task? Not in Zimbabwe. There was no diesel or gas at any of the normal stations because hyperinflation made it impossible for the stations to stay ahead of the curve. Not only were there empty shelves, there were empty gas tanks all over the country. The only way we had diesel for the hospital vehicles and generators was by using donated money to buy coupons from International Oil companies like Texaco, using U.S. Dollars. Then we could take those coupons to "special" gas stations and get the gas or diesel. It was a complicated arrangement, requiring several trips to an office in Harare to get the coupons once the money had been transferred from the U.S. I had the coupons so I was able to get diesel *as long as the station in Masvingo had it*, and that day they did. Over the previous five years, there would periodically be fuel at normal stations, and during those times it was not unusual to see cars backed up for several blocks waiting to be served. If the station ran out of fuel, the cars would sometimes stay in line for days or even weeks hoping a new supply would arrive. *Is that any way to run a country?* Finally, it was back to the police station to get my permit, and I headed home over that dusty and bumpy road that my aching back knew so well.

*

January 2009: Once again we were on our way to South Africa on Safari—only instead of hunting animals, we were hunting supplies. We had the hospital Toyota Range Rover Ambulance because of its larger capacity, plus the four-ton truck. Our "mission" was to get as many hospital supplies as possible, plus all the items needed to construct a steel tower to support three 250-gallon water tanks, along with two of the tanks. These were to be used for irrigation of the hospital gardens. I had emailed the company an order for the steel and the tanks. The other supplies would have to be scavenged by Ms Hove and the driver of the truck, Mr. Jeketera. Loretta would shop for our personal groceries and supplies.

It was only 180 miles from Masvingo to the border at Beit Bridge. Once a good blacktop road, now I had to weave my way in and around the many deep potholes. As I rounded a corner, a vehicle was stopped directly in my path. As I veered into the other lane, I hit a deep hole. We were lucky not to be thrown into the ditch or worse. I stopped to look at the tire and thought it was okay, but the farther I drove, the more I realized there was something wrong. I hoped it would get us to a garage at Louis Trichardt, about 60 miles inside South Africa. It did, but I had to buy a new tire as soon as we got there. That pothole cost me $150.

Forty miles from the border we stopped at "The Lion and The Elephant," a convenient stopping point that once was a fancy place for both eating and lodging. Now, because of so few tourists, it had fallen into disrepair. There was little in the way of food and the rooms were one star at best. Still, it had one of the few clean restroom facilities along the way, so we always stopped, used the facilities, and ordered a coke or a beer. This time I ordered cokes for everyone and we sat in the parking lot eating our lunch while watching monkeys cavorting through the Msasa trees.

Arriving at the border at 11:00 AM, we were lucky to find only a short line waiting to cross. On a recent trip, just as we got there, several buses arrived and it took hours to get through. Usually, on the South African side, things went quicker—unless the Border customs agents happened to be on "slow down." On this trip it went quickly, and we were soon through both sides of the border.

As we crossed into South Africa we immediately noticed the difference: A wide, paved, and well maintained road with no potholes; roadside stalls filled with oranges, bananas, avocado, grapefruit, green beans, corn on the cob, Coca Cola and other soft drinks; gas stations with diesel and gas at a reasonable price; green cultivated fields full of sugar cane or maize or wheat; rows upon rows of citrus trees loaded with nearly ripe fruit; and everywhere you looked, people feverishly involved in some type of commercial activity.

Just a few miles inside South Africa was the border town of Musina. It looked like any typical border town. Imagine driving across the border from the U.S. into Nogales, Mexico. Everything was available for a price—and I mean everything. From food to TVs to fridges to microwaves to girls for hire to whatever else you might want. Probably even illegal drugs—in fact, I'm quite sure you could get drugs if you knew the right contact. "Hey mister, wanta see my sister?" is a refrain heard around the world in such border towns. The free enterprise system was doing well in South Africa, whereas the controlled economy in Zimbabwe was on life support, and soon would die if they didn't do something about inflation and price controls. As I drove along, I thought, *this must be what it was like when going form East Berlin into West Berlin during the Cold War. But, the situation in Zimbabwe is even worse than it was in the Communist controlled countries. The Zimbabwe authorities have been able to outdo even the worst examples of "how to ruin an economy."*

We drove right through Musina because from past experience we knew supplies this close to the border were at least 25 percent higher than at Louis Trichardt, another 50 miles south. Along the way we continued to marvel at the lush green pastures—maize, sugarcane, beans, mango trees, orange groves, all well managed—just like Zimbabwe was a decade ago before the ill-conceived land and farm takeovers.

As we drove down from the mountaintop, we could see Louis Trichardt nestled in the green valley, with trees and houses extending like fingers away from the business district. We briefly stopped at a scenic view overlooking the town and valley. From a distance, it looked like any U. S. town sitting in a lush verdant valley. The first Dutch settlers to arrive must have thought they had found a bit heaven, with good soil, good rainfall, and plenty of sunshine—perfect for farming. Now it was a bustling community making a profit from the dire situation in Zimbabwe. At least half the vehicles had Zimbabwe license plates—all coming South to stock up on supplies. The streets were bustling with people hurrying to and fro with bundles of items no longer available in Zimbabwe. Many were entrepreneurs taking goods back to sell at a tidy profit. No matter how dire the economic situation, someone will find a way to make "a silk purse out of a sows ear."

We planned on staying two nights in a motel that had cooking facilities so we could fix most of our own meals. We had a lot to get done in the day and a half. I dropped Ms Hove and Mr. Jeketera and Loretta at the warehouse food store while I went to the bank to get a bundle of cash. The place where I was buying the steel would take a credit card, but the water tanks, pump, and maize meal needed cash, the equivalent of U.S. $5,000. That's a lot of money to be carrying around, and I wasn't happy about doing it, but had no choice. I went to Standard Bank with my passport, drivers' license, and credit card that had a $5,000 limit. They had a separate, private area of the bank for foreign exchange transactions. After waiting in line for 45 minutes, the lady clerk called me.

"I would like to get 40,000 Rand," I told her.

"Let me see your papers, including passport, another picture I.D., and the credit card you will be using."

After looking at everything, she told me, "Please have a seat. This will take some time because we have to contact your bank in the U.S." Taking all my papers and credit card and passport, she disappeared into the bowels of the bank.

An hour later, I was called back to the private cubicle and given 40,000 Rand. I placed the large bundle of cash in a money belt, strapped it under my shirt, took all my papers and left to immediately spend the cash.

I drove to pay for the tanks, then the pump, and finally to the wholesaler for the maize meal. A rush of relief washed over me to be rid of the cash. Just two months previously, two African Dominican Sisters had obtained cash in a similar manner, and a short time later in the parking lot of a large mall, they were robbed at gunpoint. Fortunately, they weren't injured, but now they didn't have the cash needed to buy supplies for their congregation. They surmised that someone at the bank had alerted the thieves about a Dominican Sister carrying a large amount of cash, so they knew who to watch and got to her when no one was around to stop them.

Next was the steel company to pay for the steel I had ordered and make sure it would be ready to load the next morning. That came to another $4,500 in U.S. dollars and was charged to my credit card—after the appropriate delay to assure the bank in the U.S. that I had properly identified myself.

I went back to get Loretta to see how the shopping was going at the warehouse. Walking into the store was a revelation after recently meandering through stores in Zimbabwe. Every aisle was stocked to the ceiling with boxes and boxes of cooking oil, soap, dish detergent, mops, hospital cleaning supplies, cases of canned food of every description, 50 pound sacks of sugar and flour and maize meal (but more expensive than at the wholesaler I was dealing with). There were large flatbed trolleys piled high with every sort of commodity, filling the aisles as people waited to check out. Some had ten or even twenty trolleys. We could hear Shona being spoken throughout the store. It looked and sounded like all of Zimbabwe was in this one store buying everything in sight.

We felt like children in a candy store at Christmas time: "Give me several of those;" "Let's get five cases of that;" "Oh, we need three boxes of those." It quickly became evident that I needed to put a limit on how much could be purchased. The truck was going to be full of steel, water tanks, and maize meal. It would likely be over the weight limit of four tons for the truck, so everything else had to fit inside the ambulance. It was starting to look like that would be problematic. I cautioned everyone about our limitations on space, and we collectively decided to leave the trolleys in line for the next day so we could go to the motel and decide what was *really* essential. Also, it had been a long day and I felt in need of a beer and supper. We left St. Theresa's at 5:00 AM and the travel, getting through the border, and now the shopping had taken its toll on all of us. We were dragging along like some rag-tag outfit in need of food and sleep. It would be the night to cook something easy at the motel, enjoy a beer, and get to bed early. The next day we attacked the stores with renewed vigor, finished the shopping and the careful loading of the vehicles, and celebrated our accomplishments by eating out.

*

Five A.M.: It was still dark and rather chilly. We wanted to be at the border by 8:00, hoping against hope there wouldn't be too long a line on the Zimbabwe side. Even the South African side could take a long time because of the wait to apply for the Value Added Tax refund. Most merchandise purchased in South Africa had a VAT of 14%. *If* you were taking the supplies out of the country, you could apply for a refund of the tax. Since we purchased such a large amount, it was worthwhile to go through the tedious process.

At 7:00 AM, still dark and about five miles from the border, a policewoman stopped us. After perusing my U.S. driver's license, she looked at the ambulance and then at the truck. She hemmed and hawed and finally said, "It looks like that truck should be weighed. It might be over the limit."

I handed her my passport with a 100 Rand note folded inside (about $10). She looked at my passport, back at the truck, handed me the passport and said, "Have a good trip." I was simply following advice from the people where I bought the steel. They warned me I would probably be stopped, but that the police were just looking for a bribe. Going through the weight station could have taken hours. *Once more, the slippery slope.*

Getting through customs on the South African side was easy *until* I went to stand in line for the VAT refund—that took two hours. I've never been a patient person, and that day I was really tested, but what could I do? It was worth several hundred dollars, and those dollars could be used the next time we shopped in South Africa.

We crossed the bridge over the muddy Limpopo River to the Zimbabwe side. As usual, there was a long line of trucks and cars waiting for Customs, but we had seen worse. This was the part of each trip I dreaded the most. I always worried that something would happen—like getting thrown in prison for bribing someone. It was nearly impossible to get through the process unless you arranged some *"help"* from one of the many men and women who assisted people through the maze of form filling, trekking from counter to counter, how much to pay, then to the next counter, then "help" with the outside customs agent and finally the person at the gate. This time, I negotiated with a man to help me.

"I have all the forms I need," I said.

"I'll help you through everything. No problem," he replied.

"How much?"

"Five hundred Rand ($50)."

"No, I'll find someone else."

"How much will you pay?"

"I'll give you 250 Rand when everything is finished."

"I need 100 right now to help pay the fees."

"O.K." and I handed him the 100 Rand note.

First we went to the vehicle window with my permit to allow the vehicles back into the country. I paid the clerk 200 million Zimbabwe dollars for the ambulance and 400 million for the truck.

*

I must backtrack and explain more about the hyper-hyperinflation. On a trip to Masvingo in late December, I went to see Joe, a friend who was manager at a large building supply business. The banking system was a total mess, but you could still transfer money between accounts and the Customs people at the border would accept my check. The government could never keep up with the daily inflationary spiral, so the Customs taxes were always seriously behind what the actual cost should have been. I knew I had to have a *lot* of money in my Zimbabwe bank account for this trip.

"Joe, how much can I get for $20?"

He called someone. Looking at me with raised eyebrows and a grin, he said, "Twenty-one trillion dollars. I can transfer it today." To put things into perspective, that means the 600 million for vehicle fees was only a fraction of one cent.

I handed him the twenty, he called his bank, and it was arranged. I was a trillionaire — richer than Bill Gates and Warren Buffett combined.

*

Next, we walked to the counter to pay duty on the supplies I purchased. I had a form from the tax people in Masvingo letting me bring most of the equipment in Duty Free since it was for the hospital, but still I had to pay for everything else. The clerk finally figured it all out and I wrote a check for eighteen billion, seven hundred and fifty-six million, four hundred and forty-two thousand, and three hundred Zimbabwe dollars—equivalent to

2 cents. For them to replace the forms I had to complete would cost many times that amount. No wonder the country was broke.

I walked out of the building with my "assistant," who now said, "I know you have all the papers, but those men over there also need to be paid something, or they'll hold you up for hours."

"Don't tell me. You think I should give you more money?"

"Unless you want to stay here for the rest of the day."

I glanced at the agents who were eying the two of us and then back at "my" man. It was obvious these men were in league with each other, so I felt he was telling the truth. "How much more?"

"500 Rand for them plus the 250 you promised me. That should do it."

Now I was in a bind. I had started this process and couldn't stop it— *once on the slippery slope, it's difficult to get off.* Reluctantly I gave him 500 Rand, and he went to talk with the agents. They stared at me a long time, but finally waved us forward, looked into both vehicles, checked the papers and stamped them, and waived us towards the exit gate. I slipped the agent his fee and heaved a sigh of relief. But it was too soon to relax.

Just as we approached that final gate, there was a man in a white suit. I have never before felt I was in the presence of evil, but this man exuded something that made my skin crawl. He was maybe 30 years old, but looked like he already had lived a rough life. He had several scars down one cheek and a couple of teeth missing. His eyes seemed to stare right through me. There was no hint of a smile. A single word to describe him would be "brutal."

"Where are you going?" he barked.

"This is all for St. Theresa Hospital in Chirumanzu District," I politely told him. He could have figured it out by himself since the ambulance and truck both had "St. Theresa Hospital" signs on each door.

He glared at me, and then at the truck with the large amount of steel and water tanks. "Let me see your passport."

I handed him my passport with the standard 100 Rand note folded inside. He looked at it, then at the truck, and back at me. With hatred in his eyes, he said, "For that load, it's not nearly enough."

Loretta heard the exchange and said, "Get his name." I knew that was exactly the wrong thing to say.

"What did you say?" he yelled.

"She didn't say anything," I said, gently waving my open palms back and forth. "I have all the papers here. I paid the Customs fees, and thought I had done everything I was supposed to do."

"What did she say?" he again roared, fiercely glaring at her.

Shaking my head back and forth and again waving my open palms as if in supplication, I said, "She didn't mean anything. I'm sorry. She didn't mean anything."

For a long time he stared at Loretta as if he could harm her just through his eyes, and it felt like he could. She cowered against the window and looked the other way. Finally, through clenched teeth he said, "For that kind of equipment, you're supposed to have a clearing agent."

"I'm sorry. I didn't know that," and I fumbled in my pocket for more Rand. Not even counting it, I handed it over. I didn't know how much it was and didn't care. I just wanted to be away from there.

Smirking, he looked at it, once again glowered at us, at the truck and back at me, and finally in a low and barely audile voice, grunted, "O.K. You can leave, but next time get a clearing agent. Do you hear me?" I meekly nodded. He acted as though he had just done us a tremendous favor—and maybe he had. With that he nodded to the young lady at the gate and she raised the barrier to let us through.

With shaking hands and a hammering heart, I wasn't sure I could drive through the gate, but somehow we made it and finally were outside the Customs area. I vowed I would never do that again. Now *I* glared at

Loretta and she meekly said, "Sorry," knowing that her comment was not helpful. Right then I decided that *if* we made another trip, I would go through Customs as you're supposed to and take my chances. No more using agents and bribes to get across, no matter how much time it might take. It just wasn't worth the worry and stress.

A few miles from the border, I had both vehicles stop so I could walk around to burn up some of the adrenalin coursing through my body.

"Who do you think that was?" I asked.

Mr. Jeketera said, "He was C.I.D. for sure." The Criminal Investigation Department is the equivalent of the Soviet KGB, with a lot of thugs operating on their own and terrorizing whomever and wherever they want.

"Do you think he was just shaking us down so he could get more money?"

"Yeah. For sure."

"I was so scared. I thought we would end up in a Beit Bridge jail and no one would know where we were."

As I drove along, I started to think of all the bright rejoinders I might have said to that jerk at the border. I would have loved to see his florid face and the scars on his cheek blossoming into bright red blotches, but then the reality hit me of being thrown into a Beit Bridge jail cell with twenty or so other miscreants, sharing a flimsy louse-infested blanket, a single bucket for a toilet and no hope of being bailed out. I realized it was good those rejoinders were kept to myself—especially since Loretta and Ms Hove would almost certainly have received a similar fate.

I couldn't believe some of the filthy things I imagined saying to him. *A Catholic Mission Doctors' representative thinking those thoughts?* Still, it helped pass the time and relieved some my stress, and before I knew it we were halfway to Masvingo. The rest of the trip was uneventful, and we were home by nightfall.

*

I thought the story of the trip was behind us, only to find it was a trip that "kept on taking and taking." Two days after returning, I downloaded my U.S. bank transactions via our satellite Internet connection, and discovered there were four unauthorized charges on my credit card. Obviously, someone at the bank had taken all my information—credit card and authorization numbers, passport number, drivers license info—and either used it themselves or gave it to someone else to buy several items: clothing; electronics; drugstore supplies; and an airplane ticket on Iberia Airlines—total charges of $2600. By the use of Skype, I talked with a fraud officer at my bank in the U.S., confirming the charges that were fraudulent. Within a couple of days, they reversed the charges and sent me a new credit card.

*

At the time, we didn't realize it but that trip was *a step along the way* in completing our missionary journey—we discovered we were getting too old for such adventures.

We made two more trips to South Africa for hospital supplies—fortunately none as exciting or frightening as the January trip—but still stressful—and in April we had a nine-day vacation. We drove to a suburb of Johannesburg to visit the Davies—good friends from Driefontein and Silveira days in the 1970's. Tony and Deirdre visited us twice at St. Theresa's, and they reciprocated with an invitation for us to stay with them. Tony and I always had animated conversations on the way forward for health care in Zimbabwe and South Africa. He was a Professor Emeritus at Witwatersrand University in the Industrial Medicine department, having been Head of the Department for many years after leaving Zimbabwe in 1982. After three nights with them, we travelled to a mountainous area near the Kruger National Park to stay at a comfortable hotel. Because it was the "off-season," the rates were reasonable and within our budget. For four days we enjoyed wonderful meals, having our every whim catered to, sleeping late, and sightseeing at our leisure. After the obligatory hospital and personal grocery shopping in Louis Trichardt, we drove the 60 miles to the border, getting across in record time and with a minimum of fuss and bother, and best of all, without any bribes.

Back at St. Theresa's it gradually became obvious to us that it was time for us to leave. One day in early May I came home for tea with Loretta, slumped into a chair on the verandah, and said, "Damn."

"What's the matter?"

"I blew up at one of the hospital workers. It was for good reason, but still I shouldn't have handled it that way."

"What happened?"

"He manages the free food we get for patients with AIDS. I have a two-year-old in pediatrics who desperately needs food. He doesn't have AIDS but still needs the food so I sent the mother to him, and he refused her. I sent a strong note, and he still sent her away. Then I sent a note for him to meet me in Ms Hove's office. I read the riot act to him, telling him in loud and rather profane terms that I was in charge and he would do as I said or he could find a new job."

"Sounds like he needed telling off."

"He did, but not the way I did it. It seems the littlest thing sets me off and I don't like it."

"I'm sorry."

"Yes, I know." I stopped to take a sip of tea, looked at her and said, "I think maybe we should go back for good this summer rather than waiting another year."

She got up, put her arms around my shoulders and said, "Yes, I've been thinking that too. It's been hard for me because I'm not able to help people as much as I used to since the hospital needs all the donations we receive. Also, I'm worried about the bouts of back and hip pain I've been having."

Just like the decision in Colorado in 1969 when we clearly heard a call to do missionary work, we now heard an equally clear call that said, "It's time to go home."

The following week, I invited Sister Andrea to tea, telling her I had some important news. Loretta wanted me to "ease my way into the topic," but since I have always handled difficult issues head-on, after pouring tea and offering Andrea a piece of Loretta's carrot cake, I said, "You know, as we get older, it has become more and more difficult for us to put up with the daily frustrations and hardships. Loretta and I feel that it's time for us to go home to our family. We plan to leave in July."

Her head jerked up and with an almost frightened look, she said, "What's happened? Has someone said something or done something to upset you?"

"No, nothing like that. We are both having some health issues and feel the time has come for us to go back and be with our family and for me to really retire. We have a strong feeling that it's time to go."

"Have you told anyone else?"

"Not yet. We'll invite Dr. Murungu and Ms Hove to tea tomorrow and tell them and they can let everyone else know. You can tell the other Sisters today, but otherwise keep it quiet until tomorrow."

"I can't believe it. What will we do?"

"You'll do just fine. The goal of all missionaries should be to work themselves out of a job, and I honestly feel that's what we've done."

"No one will be able to do what you two have done."

"It's kind of you to say that, but you know as well as I that at some point Zimbabwean doctors need to step in and do the work, just as you Zimbabwean Sisters have stepped into leadership roles in the Dominican organization."

"Maybe so, but it won't be the same."

Once the decision was made, the rest was easy: Decide what we wanted to take to the U.S.; what to do with "our things" in the house; what would happen to our maid and gardener; who would take our cat. I promised to return for three or four weeks every year for "a few years," just to keep in touch and to make sure things were going well (and they were).

The women of Loretta's prayer group had a party for her at our teahouse in late June. They arrived in their best clothes. Monica, our maid, killed and cleaned a chicken that was cooked by the ladies, along with sadza and vegetables. The table was set with a fancy tablecloth and our best dishes. After the meal, Monica served cake with ice cream. The dessert was followed with dancing and drumming and singing as each of the women offered a small gift of a woven basket or table matt or embroidered cloth, and they tearfully said goodbye to Loretta.

Of course, there had to be a traditional "Good-bye Party" with the entire hospital staff. The student nurses produced a skit that seriously roasted me—I might have been offended if it hadn't been so accurate. One of the male student nurses, wearing a white coat and a stethoscope around his neck, haughtily strolled into the ward and started barking orders: "Why aren't you ready for rounds? You know I always want to start on time. Where are the student nurses? Come on, let's go. Time's wasting," and he rapidly started pushing a bed-table towards the first patient.

Several student nurses gathered around.

"Nurse, what's wrong with this patient?"

"Uh, Uh, Uh."

"Spit it out nurse. Don't you know this patient?"

Meekly, "Yes doctor. She has T.B. and is on treatment for it."

"Well, why didn't you say that in the first place?"

"Sorry doctor."

"Let's go to the next patient. What's wrong with her?"

Second student nurse, "She has HIV and is starting on treatment today."

"What's her blood count?"

Picking up the chart and peering through it, she said, "Let me see."

"I don't want you to SEE it; I want you to KNOW it."

And on it went. Sometimes it's painful to see yourself through the eyes of others. I had to remind myself that by nature students are irreverent and critical. Still, it was funny and was balanced by the more traditional speeches that followed.

Finally it was time for me to say "Thank You" to the staff. The words stuck in my throat as I stood there with tears running down my cheeks, a kaleidoscope of thoughts flashing through my mind of the many people who made our time at St. Theresa's so meaningful: *Gift, the small orphan boy who briefly brought joy and tears to our home; Finance Mutero, the first of our staff to start on AIDS treatment, who was brave enough to face up to the community stigma; Monica, the woman who doubled her weight in one year of treatment, going from cadaver-like to a picture of health; Eric, the man who was paralyzed but gradually regained the use of his legs and acted as though he had won the lottery as I watched him sit on a tree stump in front of his hut, with no electricity, no water, no heat, but joy radiating from his face; Florence, my faithful and ever-smiling interpreter and surgical assistant who used her meager salary to support several family members; the Cavanaugh's, good friends and compatriots; Sister Andrea, indefatigably providing loving care to so many dying of AIDS and providing support for AIDS orphans; Doctor Murungu who stayed for five years giving loving medical care to his people; Ms Hove and Elizabeth, who together provided administrative stability in times of financial instability . . .*

I gathered myself and tearfully expressed our gratitude to the staff for their good work and the cooperation they had given over the previous eight years. Most of those years had been financially difficult for them, especially when there was no salary for months at a time because the government ran out of money. Some of the most "missionary-like" people we met were not missionaries at all—they were simply hospital staff that continued to do praiseworthy work under strenuous conditions.

The morning we left, the entire staff convened in front of the hospital for a final farewell. We walked around the large circle of friends, giving handshakes and hugs, tears unashamedly running down our cheeks. At last, climbing into the car and waving a last goodbye, we slowly drove down the dusty road, through the Township to the blacktop road, and on to Harare. Another sad farewell with many friends in Harare, and the next day—July 4th, 2009—we boarded a South African Airways jet, destination Orlando, Florida—exactly 39 years to the day since we first arrived in Rhodesia.

We had come "full circle." *Our Missionary steps were complete as we travelled to a new home in the U.S., forever changed by our experiences in Rhodesia and Zimbabwe, pondering where the next steps might lead. Just like when we made the decision in 1969, we felt the presence of Christopher, forever two, forever our own Angel looking after us, forever . . .*